Wider than the Sky

Literature and Medicine
MARTIN KOHN AND CAROL DONLEY, EDITORS

Wider than the Sky

Essays and Meditations on the Healing Power of Emily Dickinson

Edited by

Cindy MacKenzie & Barbara Dana

The Kent State University Press

KENT, OHIO

© 2007 by The Kent State University Press, Kent, Ohio 44242
Library of Congress Catalog Card Number 2007021852
ISBN 978-0-87338-919-8
Manufactured in the United States of America

11 10 09 08 07   5 4 3 2 1

The poems of Emily Dickinson are reprinted by permission of the publishers and Trustees of Amherst College from *The Poems of Emily Dickinson: Variorum Edition,* Ralph W. Franklin, ed., Cambridge, Mass.: The Belknap Press of Harvard University Press, Copyright © 1998 by the President and Fellows of Harvard College. Copyright © 1951, 1955, 1979 by the President and Fellows of Harvard College.

The letters of Emily Dickinson are reprinted by permission of the publishers from *The Letters of Emily Dickinson,* Thomas H. Johnson, ed., Cambridge, Mass.: The Belknap Press of Harvard University Press, Copyright © 1958, 1986, the President and Fellows of Harvard College; 1914, 1924, 1932, 1942 by Martha Dickinson Bianchi; 1952 by Alfred Leete Hampson; 1960 by Mary L. Hampson.

Quotations from the original manuscript pages of the following poems by Emily Dickinson are reprinted by permission of The Houghton Library, Harvard University © The President and Fellows of Harvard College: "After a great pain, a formal feeling comes" *MS Am 1118.3 (26c);* "Surgeons must be very careful" *MS Am 1118.3 (7g);* "Pain has an Element of Blank" *MS Am 1118.3 (52b);* "I dwell in Possibility" *MS Am 1118.3 (106a);* "Revolution is the Pod Systems rattle from" *MS Am 1118.3 (190c);* "Pain expands the Time" *MS Am 1118.3 (211c);* "Much Madness is divinest Sense" *MS Am 1118.3 (151d);* "A little Madness in the Spring" *MS Am 1118.3 (229).*

"Thunder Road" by Bruce Springsteen. Copyright © 2003 by Bruce Springsteen (ASCAP). Reprinted by permission. International copyright secured. All rights reserved.

LIBRARY OF CONGRESS CATALOGING-IN-PUBLICATION DATA
Wider than the sky : essays and meditations on the healing power of Emily Dickinson / edited by Cindy MacKenzie and Barbara Dana.
    p.   cm. — (Literature and medicine ; no. 11)
Includes bibliographical references and index.
ISBN 978-0-87338-953-2 (cloth : alk. paper) ∞
ISBN 978-0-87338-919-8 (pbk. : alk. paper) ∞
1. Dickinson, Emily, 1830–1886—Criticism and interpretation. 2. Mind and body in literature. 3. Reading—Psychological aspects. 4. Poetry—Therapeutic use. I. MacKenzie, Cindy. II. Dana, Barbara.
PS1541.Z5W54 2007
811'.4—dc22   2007021852

British Library Cataloging-in-Publication data are available.

For Emily Dickinson and all my healers
C. M.

For Timothy Vernon
B. D.

Contents

Preface

Barbara Dana

In the summer of 2002 I went to Amherst to attend my first conference of the Emily Dickinson International Society—sixty scholars and me! I was working on a novel based on the young life of my favorite poet, and although I had not yet begun the actual writing, I had been immersed in research for over two years. I'd been reading the poems, the letters, the biographies, and the essays, as well as making many trips to Amherst. I had spent long hours in Emily's garden, her bedroom, her parlor, and at her gravesite. I had been to Harvard to see her bureau (the one in which she kept her poems) and her small writing desk, hardly large enough for such a grand outpouring. I saw the piano she so loved and a sampler she made when she was ten. I viewed a collection of several of the original manuscripts being housed at Harvard on a temporary basis. At the Frost Library at Amherst College I saw a lock of her hair, which looked like spun gold, and her Latin book, shared with Abby Wood, complete with a spunky comment in the margin of page 12 ("Due Monday—How mean!") and a drawing of a man with a large nose and a serious expression whom I took to be the professor of Emily's Latin course. I spent days in the archives at the Jones Library pouring over seemingly endless amounts of material, including letters written by Emily's father, transcripts of sermons given by Philadelphia minister Charles Wadsworth, records of medical prescriptions ordered by the Dickinson family from the local pharmacy, and articles on tuberculosis, Bright's disease, conditions of the eyes, hypertension, lupus, anxiety disorders, and depression, along with records of the eye doctor in Boston who treated Emily for a mysterious eye condition. I walked her school-day route to Amherst Academy, the location of which had become a parking lot with a plaque marking the spot where the school once stood. I visited Mount Holyoke College, where she spent much of her seventeenth year. On North Pleasant Street I stopped by the Mobil gas station that had so irreverently replaced the home the poet had lived in for fifteen years, from age nine to twenty-four. A particularly enjoyable part of my research was the exploration into the habits, personality, and appearance of Newfoundland dogs. I attended dog shows, interviewed owners, and met several of these huge, bearlike creatures, getting to know the lumbering, lifesaving breed, one of which was Emily's beloved Carlo. Emily was in my blood.

But I was not a scholar. My fields were acting and fiction writing. I felt decidedly out of place at the conference. These people had immersed themselves in all aspects of Dickinson's poetry and letters and had written dissertations about things like cognitive linguistics, phenomenology, and synaesthesia. At conferences they presented papers with such titles as "Amplitude of Queer Desire in Dickinson's Erotic Language" and "Dickinson at the Limits of Philology." They wrote books on things like "the significance of the dash in Dickinson's poetry from 1861 to 1865." They knew what they were talking about. I only felt it.

Notebook in hand, back straight, mind alert, I quietly kept to myself. Several pleasant scholars introduced themselves, welcoming me to the conference, but I was intimidated. The only question I dared ask was if anyone knew where Carlo used to sleep. No one seemed to know. After one of the workshops I got to talking with a smart, attractive woman with a disarming sense of humor. She didn't know where Carlo slept but asked if I had been to Zanna's, a clothing shop down the street from the renowned Mobil gas station. I said I had and mentioned having almost bought a pair of boots that had caught my eye. The conversation went from there to feeling comfortable in one's clothing, to the joy of feeling attractive, to men, and to divorce, an experience both of us had unfortunately shared. The woman's name was Cindy MacKenzie. She had edited the invaluable *Concordance to the Letters of Emily Dickinson* and was now considering working on a book about Dickinson's power to console. The poet had helped her through an intense period of pain, and she felt others might also have experienced that same healing power.

I was one of them. I had started working on my Dickinson novel during the breakup of my marriage of thirty-five years. Emily had helped me through the time when I thought I would die, or was dead already, or hoped I soon would be.

The conference continued. Another talk began, and another, and soon it was four o'clock, with free time until a cocktail reception at five-thirty. I was thinking about Zanna's and how there would be time to stop by there and check out the boots and still get back to the hotel for a quick shower before the reception. So off I went. When I got to the store Cindy was inside trying on a colorful unstructured jacket that looked as if it had been made for her. She greeted me and asked if I liked the jacket, and even more importantly, if I would be interested in working on the Dickinson healing edition with her. I answered yes to both questions.

We quickly saw that our coming from two entirely different directions in the study of Dickinson would work in a new and interesting way for the book. We envisioned essays from a wide range of readers, not merely scholars but artists, writers, poets, psychologists, and others. Some essays would be personal. Others would be scholarly. Some might combine the two approaches (as Cindy's essay accomplishes), giving the edition a unique texture as well as wide appeal.

Cindy knew many scholars, familiar to her from her academic background, whom she could invite, and I knew many actors and writers who might want to contribute. I immediately thought of asking Julie Harris. I had known Julie for years. Now a treasured friend, she had been my idol since I was a young girl. She introduced me to Emily Dickinson more than thirty years ago when I saw her brilliant performance in *The Belle of Amherst.* I knew she was devoted to the poet. Another actor-friend, Anne Jackson, had been doing spirited readings of Dickinson's poetry for years. I would ask her. I knew that Maurice Sendak had long been inspired by Dickinson. He had mentioned the fact to my son, Anthony, when they worked on a project together in New York. I thought of Gregory Orr's insightful chapter on Dickinson in his book *Poetry as Survival,* of Richard Wilbur's vivid poem about Emily, of Joyce Carol Oates's words in the introduction to her collection of favorite Dickinson poems. And I thought of Marion Woodman. Dr. Woodman had been there with me, along with Emily, during the intense pain of my divorce. Her books helped me enormously. I kept a copy of *Leaving My Father's House* on my bedside table for over a year. Later, I heard her incredible tape *Emily Dickinson and the Demon Lover,* in which she refers to Emily as her "soul poet." I knew we must try to reach her and ask if she would consider contributing. And I had other ideas. Biographer Polly Longsworth had written several books about Emily that had touched me deeply. A mutual friend, writer Shulamith Oppenheim, had introduced me to Polly, who had provided endless information and welcome support. A new friend, poet/professor Joy Ladin, had also been tremendously helpful during my writing process by spending many long hours going over the poems with me and bringing me closer to the poet through her work. "I would ask my new friend," I thought.

And so it went: scholars, writers, actors, poets, weavers, ministers, psychologists, and others all gathered together to share their experiences and perspectives on the healing power of Emily Dickinson. I am grateful to all of them.

Cindy and I have many to thank for their help in making *Wider than the Sky* a reality. I want to thank Julie Harris, my constant inspiration; Judith Schmidt for her endless support and love; Shulamith Oppenheim for the introductions and the encouragement; children's book author/editor Charlotte Zolotow for her belief in me and for sharing her love of Dickinson; our editor, Joanna Hildebrand Craig, for her invaluable help and encouragement; prominent EDIS member, writer/professor Jane Donahue Eberwein, for her generosity and enthusiasm for the project; director of Interpretation and Programming at the Emily Dickinson Museum, Cindy Dickinson, always so helpful and welcoming; my daughter-in-law, Pamela, for bringing Emily to my attention when I most needed her; and, of course, Emily—for being herself.

Introduction

CINDY MACKENZIE

From the time I first read a selection of Emily Dickinson's poems in an undergraduate class, I felt their power in a way that parallels the way in which Dickinson herself described her criteria for recognizing poetry: "If I read a book [and] it makes my whole body feel so cold no fire can ever warm me I know *that* is poetry. If I feel physically as if the top of my head were taken off, I know *that* is poetry. These are the only way I know it. Is there any other way" (L342a). Dickinson's poetry makes me feel in ways that not only comfort but also disturb me, that appeal strongly not only to my emotions but just as strongly to my intellect. Most importantly, because her poetry provokes me, it also has the capacity to change me. At that time, however, I had no idea that her lines, even her individual words, were becoming an integral part of my own psyche, a rich source of nourishment, real things, objects to hold onto during troubling times, to turn over in my mind, and to repeat to myself whenever I needed fortitude. In my own essay in this collection, I explain how Dickinson's poetry became a lifeline for me during an emotionally difficult time and how she lead me, through her poetry and letters, to a fuller, more creative, and authentic life. Through my work on Dickinson, now going on over twenty years, I have pursued both a personal and intellectual longing and have found much fulfillment in this singular poet's work. My feelings of gratitude and indebtedness to Emily Dickinson and her rich legacy motivated me to share my story along with those of others whose love for this poet also offered them comfort and hope in the face of life's challenges.

I met these kindred spirits in various ways. First, at the Emily Dickinson International Society (EDIS) meetings, I had discussions about the theme of healing many years ago with contributors Joan Kirkby and Cynthia Hogue, both of whom had suffered severe physical and emotional pain and who agreed with me that it would be a worthy project. I then met Lois Kauffman (who did not submit an essay) at a Dickinson meeting in St. Paul. Her grief over a lost daughter, killed in an automobile accident, was painfully fresh and clearly reflected in her face. That she could find solace for such an unbearable wound by reading

Dickinson's poetry confirmed for me the extent of the poet's healing powers. Lois's gratitude to Emily Dickinson, her deep insights into the poetry, and her ongoing work with families who have lost a child have touched all of us within the Dickinson Society who have heard her story. I met two others, Brian Clark and JoAnn Orr, in cyberspace, but they could not be more real to me than if I had met them on the street. Their belief in this project bolstered my desire to make publication a reality. I am grateful for all their suggestions and support and, of course, their friendship. Brian's vast reading, strong intellect, and unending creativity make him an extraordinarily fine reader, and I have relied on his responses to many of my ideas. Like Dickinson, Brian likes to provoke; in fact, I think he *has* to provoke and question. He has pushed me to consider new ways of thinking by compelling me to enlarge my reading and my intellect. We owe to him the fittingly beautiful title of this collection. JoAnn Orr, a graphic designer and owner/manager of Morning Glory Greetings in Grand Rapids, Michigan, whose generously donated Emily Dickinson magnets adorn the refrigerators of those who have visited the Emily Dickinson Homestead gift shop in Amherst, is an energetic and intelligent reader who has also been consoled and strengthened by Dickinson's work. Emily Dickinson became an important part of her life after the early accidental death of her husband. Her insightful reading of the poet currently extends beyond the letters and poems to anything she can find that is connected to the poet's writing or life. JoAnn has a remarkable collection of old editions, anthologies, and newspaper clippings found over many years in bookstores and antique stores. For all her ideas, especially those that have been incorporated into this book, for her support, and mostly for her friendship, I am deeply grateful.

At a meeting in Amherst, Massachusetts, in the summer of 2002, I first met and talked with my coeditor, Barbara Dana, about our connection to Emily Dickinson. We immediately felt connected by our interest in and genuine love for this incomparable nineteenth-century poet. As we continued to get to know each other, we soon discovered that we were personally drawn to the poet because of the way she had helped each of us through the difficult experience of divorce. We both knew of many others who felt the same way. Therefore, our aim in bringing together this collection of reminiscences, tributes, and personal and scholarly essays from such a wide and varied group of contributors is to highlight the personal impact of Dickinson's words on all kinds of readers and especially to bear witness to the significant consolatory power of the poet's work. While there is an enormous amount of scholarly work on Dickinson, we wanted to open the discussion to an even wider reading audience by including highly subjective readings that can often get lost in academic circles. Since each of us came to the poet from a different perspective—mine, scholarly; Barbara's, through the performing arts—we were fascinated by and truly appreciative of the rich manner in which we complemented each other's readings. Similarly, while the scholarly contributors appreciate the opportunity to express their personal devotion to the poet, the nonscholars appreciated the opportunity to express their thoughts and feelings in a more formal context. Just as Dickinson allies both the power of intense feeling and profound wisdom in her words, we were pleased to promote a bridge between the theoretical insights of scholarly essays and the highly subjective perceptions of personal readings, believing that one can nourish the other.

Along with our own essays, we have invited many well-known names in Dickinson scholarship—Cynthia Hogue, Joy Ladin, Polly Longsworth, Ellen Louise Hart, Martha Nell Smith, Joan Kirkby, and EDIS Distinguished Service Award recipient Roland Hagenbüchle. In addition, we have included personal tributes to the poet written by celebrated Jungian analyst and author Marion Woodman, who found in Dickinson a profound "soul connection" and a "friend" who, she believes, did nothing less than save her life. Ellen Bacon, the widow of Pulitzer award–winning composer Ernst Bacon, writes a moving testimony of her beloved husband's legacy of love inspired by the poet. Freelance writer Linda Richard shares her grief over the death of her son through a poem she composed to commemorate him. Brief testimonials include remarks from actors Julie Harris and Ann Jackson, illustrator Maurice Sendak, poet Richard Wilbur, and author Joyce Carol Oates. Acting as the poet herself in *The Belle of Amherst,* Julie Harris was never bored with the role. Dickinson's poetry continues to amaze her. Who would have imagined that illustrator Maurice Sendak keeps a small edition of Dickinson in his breast pocket so that he can find fortitude before taking on any challenge? Intriguing contributions also come from plane crash survivor Mell McDonnell, coordinator of the Colorado Shakespeare Festival, who clung to Dickinson's words "Hope is the thing with Feathers" during the descent of United Airlines 232 in 1989. Weaver Susan Hess expresses her journey of healing through the dimension of visual art inspired by the poems, and Bruce Bode, a Unitarian minister, developed a series of sermons arising from Dickinson's poems, one of which is pertinently titled "If I can stop one Heart from breaking."

The implications of Dickinson's healing powers extend far beyond the scope of this book. Marine lieutenant colonel Jim Chartier, a former English major, told a reporter from *USA Today* how he recited Dickinson's "Because I could not stop for Death" after a fateful military attack in which four men drowned in a tank.[1] Back home in California, Chartier now cares for returning casualties of war and their grieving families. In the February 2002 issue of *O, The Oprah Magazine*, Oprah Winfrey herself uses Dickinson's well-known phrase "dwell in Possibility" to discuss the "sacred privilege" of choosing one's own path.[2] And in the *New York Times Magazine*, the former U.S. senator from Nebraska Bob Kerrey spoke of his intense feelings of shame, guilt, and pain for having bombed civilians during a military operation "one awful night in Thanh Phong" in Vietnam. On an easel in his Capitol Hill office, where he sometimes painted, wrote poetry, and made newspaper collages, Kerrey had written Dickinson's painfully true line "Remorse is Memory awake" in the center of one of his watercolor paintings.[3]

Each of the contributors to this volume feels such a profound kinship to Emily Dickinson that we inevitably feel a kinship with each other. The blend of this wide expression of gratitude to the poet is testament to the enduring power of her artistic legacy and her stated "business" of love. All the essays are united by the way in which each contributor finds hope, comfort, courage, and inspiration in Emily Dickinson's work.

While it is not necessary to read this collection in sequence, the essays are loosely organized according to the development of the theme of healing. A scholarly essay is followed by a personal essay or testimonial or by a short reflection written by well-known readers. We have organized these essays beginning with those that offer illuminating contextual information about the theme. Polly Longsworth's essay begins the book because her analysis of the poet's letters clearly reveals the poet's intent to offer consolation through her work. Gregory Orr continues the discussion by explaining the lyric tradition and the universal intimacy of the confessional style that makes Dickinson's work a part of that genre. Joy Ladin finds inspiration and understanding through teaching Dickinson's phenomenological poems on death to an elderly widow who had been reading those poems with her husband in the weeks leading up to his death.

My own essay investigates the psychological process by which the poet became acclimated to painful experiences, a process that can be internalized by the reader. Cynthia Hogue and Martha Nell Smith share traumatic memories of physical suffering survived through the poet's profound insights into pain. Hogue's essay includes several of her own poems inspired by Dickinson. In an essay that includes lines from many contemporary poets as well as from Dickinson, Ellen Hart deals with the question of how poetry can help citizens cope with the trauma of September 11, 2001. Barbara Dana relates a highly personal account of her journey of healing while researching and writing a book about the poet's young life. Drawing on Freud's essay "Mourning and Melancholia" and Derrida's *The Work of Mourning,* Joan Kirkby comes to terms with the grief of bereavement in an illuminating and powerful essay that finds Dickinson to be the reader's "philosophical friend."

Because of the highly subjective nature of the collection, we editors felt it was very important to allow each author to quote from his or her preferred edition of the poems. We have, therefore, indicated the edition used in a citation that appears in an unnumbered footnote on the first page of each chapter. Throughout the chapter's text, however, we have included the conventional numbering of Dickinson's poems, placing the Johnson (J) edition number first and then the Franklin (Fr). Also, references to the Manuscript edition are indicated with *MB*; references to Dickinson's letters are noted by *L,* and the numbers correspond to any of the Johnson editions published by the Belknap Press of Harvard University Press. The Index to Poems Cited is also arranged by the Johnson/Franklin numbering, regardless of the edition used by the contributor.

Notes

1. Elliot Blair Smith, "The Road to Baghdad," *USA Today,* April 7, 2004.
2. Oprah Winfrey, "This Month's Mission," *O, The Oprah Magazine,* February 2002.
3. Gregory L. Vistica, "One Awful Night in Thanh Phong," *New York Times Magazine,* April 25, 2002.
4. Richard B. Sewall, *The Life of Emily Dickinson* (Cambridge, Mass.: Harvard Univ. Press, 1998), 689–90.

Overleaf: "If I can stop one heart from breaking" (J919/F982), *The Manuscript Books of Emily Dickinson,* ed. R. W. Franklin (Cambridge, Mass.: Belknap Press of Harvard University Press, 1981), 2:1198. Page reprinted by permission of The Houghton Library, Harvard University *MS Am 1118.3* (178e) © The President and Fellows of Harvard College.

If I can stop One
Heart from breaking
I shall not live
in vain
If I can ease One
Life the Aching
Or cool One Pain

Or help One fainting
Robin
Unto his Nest again
I shall not live
in vain

———————

"The Might of Human love"
Emily Dickinson's Letters of Healing

Polly Longsworth

In the autumn of 1884, when the impulsive Helen Hunt Jackson, then a popular American author, urged Emily Dickinson to appoint her as posthumous editor of the "portfolios of verses" that she suspected her reclusive friend of hoarding, Jackson leaned on their shared childhood in Amherst to advance her plea. "It is a cruel wrong to your 'day & generation' that you will not give them light," Jackson wrote of the assumed portfolios, and "I do not think we have a right to with hold from the world a word or a thought any more than a *deed,* which might help a single soul" (L937a). She knew that her childhood Sunday school classmate would catch her reference to the Sermon on the Mount, the hint at Christ's admonition against hiding one's God-given light under a bushel rather than letting it shine before men.[1]

In his notes concerning Jackson's proposal, Thomas H. Johnson, the editor of *The Letters of Emily Dickinson,* observes that "ED's reply to this letter pointedly ignores the request to be made literary executor," a remark that until now has gone unchallenged (937a, notes). When Jackson died the following summer, predeceasing Dickinson by nine months, the issue of editorship became moot. Today, Jackson's proposal to be made the agent for Dickinson's publication is usually cited to highlight Jackson's recognition of Dickinson's genius or to note the reclusive poet's curious stonewalling of Jackson's presumptive interest in her poems.

But Johnson's assertion that Dickinson ignored her friend's request must be reexamined, for Ralph Franklin, who reedited *The Poems of Emily Dickinson* in 1998, indicates that Johnson misread as verse a prose line in Dickinson's letter of reply (L937). In so doing, he apparently misapprehended the short poem at the end of Dickinson's promptly penciled response to Jackson's inquiry.

All citations of Dickinson's poems used in this chapter are from *The Poems of Emily Dickinson,* ed. R. W. Franklin, 3 vols. (Cambridge, Mass.: Harvard Univ. Press, 1998).

In other Motes,
Of other Myths
Your requisition be.
The Prism never held the Hues,
It only heard them play — (J1602/Fr1664)[2]

The first three lines of the poem acknowledge Jackson's petition that, "If such a thing should happen as that I should outlive you, I wish you would make me your literary legatee & executor." Dickinson's poem covertly says, Your application is "on file" and awaiting the outcome of our lives. The last two lines of the poem counter Jackson's suggestion that the poet has hidden her light under a bushel and instead present her vision of the poet, who, by nature, cannot withhold but only refract the light/word/truth that comes from God.

The self-abnegation inherent in the concept of the poet as prism is consistent with other statements Dickinson made about her role as a conduit or transmitter: "The Poets light but lamps — / Themselves — go out —" (J883/Fr930) and "Thought belong to Him who gave it — / Then — to Him Who bear / It's Corporeal illustration —" (J709/Fr788). There is sufficient evidence that Dickinson came to sense herself as God's instrument, that she recognized her extraordinary talent to be His gift, and that she saw her vocation, her ordained part, to be the passing on, the transmission, of His word, His received Truth, to the human hearts surrounding her—as she phrased it, "a privilege so awful" (J505/Fr348). For while her own faith often wavered and her personal account with God and church doctrine seems never to be finally squared, Dickinson took far more seriously than Jackson suspected the charge of bringing comforting words to the grieving, and healing insights to the brokenhearted. A central part of her work was the reception and rerouting of His consolations to those who suffered.

Although this poet's personal, individualized manner of sharing her poetry during her lifetime was far more restricted than that of the well-published Jackson, Dickinson was scarcely parsimonious with her verse. Franklin lists some 650 poems, over a third of her canon (and many more poems than Jackson wrote), that were privately sent to some four dozen recipients, friends whose joys and tribulations she sought to enhance or lighten over the years (*Poems*, app. 7). "*My* business is to love," she explained in relaying her sympathies to dear ones, "*My* business is to *sing*" (L269). There were surely more poems and more recipients than we know of involved in her acts of dispensing consolation, the adjunct industry to her work of writing poetry. Her business involved extracting from the inner and outer worlds, from nature and from consciousness, and from her own painful and joyous experiences of living, those signs and messages emblematic of God's existence, purpose, and design.

There is little doubt, from clues accumulating during a lifetime of deferral, that Dickinson anticipated and intended that the range of her light should shine with enlarged circumference after her death, by way of the posthumous publication of her work. Perhaps the largest clue to these intentions, easily overlooked and nearly neglected because it is so apparent, is that some of the most glorious poems she wrote, such as "Wild nights — Wild nights!" (J249/Fr269), "There's a certain Slant of light" (J258/Fr320), and "I dwell in Possibility —" (J657/Fr466), she shared with no one. These, along with her most anguished *cris de cœur* and the extraordinary love poems, remained hidden away among the two-thirds of her canon awaiting transmission to the world after she was gone. Meantime, however, they provided the evidence and the pretext for her mission as consoler.

> Unto a broken heart
> No other one may go
> Without the high prerogative
> Itself hath suffered too. (J1704/Fr1745)[3]

The power that she gleaned from that prerogative was exercised not through poetry alone but through such forms as flowers, puddings, and the remarkable letters that she sent to fellow sufferers. Over a thousand letters written throughout her life (and these but a sample of the many more that don't survive) exhibit Dickinson's concern for a great range of crises, contingencies, and disappointments confronting loved ones, from wayward packages or illness to misplaced trust or affection. Most particularly, she raised to high art the letters written to console relatives, friends, and neighbors who had experienced the death of a loved one. Her published correspondence includes some sixty surviving letters of solace for the human trauma that she herself found hardest to comprehend or to bear.

While no one in the nineteenth century was protected from the harsh reality of death, which struck frequently and with an immediacy scarcely familiar to us today, the poet's own exposure to its ravages occurred at somewhat of a remove. During her girlhood she lost three grandparents and her dear cousin Sophia Holland. While she was in her late teens and early twenties, several friends died of tuberculosis, and later her beloved Aunt Lavinia succumbed to the same disease. The casualties of the Civil War weighed heavily on her heart as public anguish was added to her own considerable private turmoil of the period. Still, she experienced no death within her immediate family, beneath her own roof, until her father died in June of 1874, when she was forty-three. Before that date, the consolations that she adopted were those she gleaned while growing up—derived from vivid sermons, instructive hymns, and the pious texts of her religious lessons; from books and detailed deathbed descriptions in newspaper obituaries; and from the provocative experience of living for many years next door to the town burying ground.

The first of two key concepts of consolation inherent in the Congregational faith centered on being "willing to die" (L153). A Christian departing life was expected to accept God as the Savior, voluntarily giving up this world and consigning his or her soul to its reception in the next. While privately terrified at such a prospect, Dickinson always felt reassured by knowing that a dear deceased had taken the imperative step. It lay behind her intense interest in deathbed details, as when, in 1853, troubled and uncertain about the final earthly moments of her friend Benjamin Franklin Newton, she wrote his Worcester minister, the Reverend Edward Everett Hale, to ask, "Please Sir, to tell me if he was willing to die, and if you think him at Home" (L153). In Amherst it was scandalous if someone died with "no hope," as local physician Dr. Timothy Gridley had in 1852. A quarter-century later, in 1878, Dickinson worried after his death about the immortal soul of her beloved heretic Samuel Bowles.[4]

The second Congregational consolation, which followed from the first, was the expectation of reunion with loved ones in heaven. Heaven was the reward of believers, the place where one day all pain of parting would be erased and love restored. The departed had gone ahead to "prepare the way" for those still living and were far happier there. "I would not call her back" was a common utterance. "I trust she is now in heaven & though I shall never forget her, yet I shall meet her in heaven" (L11), Emily wrote of her cousin and childhood schoolmate Sophia Holland, who died at thirteen. To such reassuring themes Dickinson added touches of her own as she matured—sometimes angels, more often birds, whose sweet music, to her mind, comforted those left behind to mourn.

These childhood consolations served Dickinson into her forties. It wasn't until the death of her father in June 1874, a shock so devastating, so unnerving and mysterious, that the tenor of the poet's understanding shifted to a new key and she abandoned some well-worn devices of her inherited faith. From the personal trauma of Edward Dickinson's lonely apoplectic fit in a Boston boarding house, she took a marked new command, amazed to find that "one who only said 'I am sorry' helped me the most when father ceased — it was too soon for language" (L730). Consolations she extended thereafter were of her own origin rather than those of the church, as when her entire message to the grieving family of Professor Snell read, "I had a father once" (L474).[5]

In seeking to ease for others the burden of pain caused by death, Dickinson's letters grew more poignant even as they grew more abstract. "To have lived is a Bliss so powerful — we must die — to adjust it," she wrote her neighbor Professor Richard Mather when his wife died in 1877, "but when you have strength to remember that Dying dispels nothing which was firm before, you have avenged sorrow —" (L523). She began, too, to embed poems in some of her letters of consolation, enhancing the potency of her message, as in these breathtaking lines of 1881 in letter 641 to her friend Thomas Wentworth Higginson, who had lost an infant daughter: "A Dimple in the Tomb / Makes that ferocious Room / A Home —" (J1489/Fr1522).

A sample of Dickinson's earlier healing work occurs in a little-known letter that she wrote in the spring of 1862 to her grieving uncle Joel Warren Norcross, the youngest brother of Emily's mother.[6] Joel, but nine years older than the poet, was a favorite relative of the Dickinson children while growing up. Dickinson lovers best know him by a spirited composition Emily sent him when he first started in business in Boston in 1850 (L29). Having prospered and become the father of two small children, Joel was forty when his wife of eight years, Lamira Jones Norcross, died unexpectedly on May 4, 1862. Dickinson's letter of condolence induces comfort by masterfully guiding Joel's thoughts from Mira's beloved face to her reunion in heaven with friends, introducing evidence of God's design from nature (here, singing birds), and ending with the soft parting of a child's goodnight. She further places his loss and grief within the generalized suffering induced by the Civil War before ending with the metaphor of Mira's absence as a journey.

> Will it comfort my sorrowing Uncle, to know that Emily, cares? Words mean very little, when the face is gone, that made our lifetime sweet — yet it grieves me so — I thought my low "I'm sorry" — would not burden you —
> When our great Rest is taken — the little pillows friends can bring, cool a weary head —
> I did'nt know dear Mira, so well as the other Nieces, knew her — but I was always thinking to, when she came next time — "next summer" — and now, I cant believe my opportunity is done —
> She was'nt so far from Nellie Converse — as she supposed — when she talked with me, and sobbed like a child, whose schoolmate had been stolen —
> Nor so far from the other Aunt — snatched like herself, in spring — I do

not think the Birds, mind our going to sleep. I notice they sing louder
— They may know Heaven — better than we — down here — so far away
— and sing so — for our sakes — I am glad Mira was not afraid — That
will always be comforting to you — and that you were with her — and
that she could talk with you —and that Mrs Wood — and Etta, were there
— to make her Good night pleasant — as among sweet neighbor's faces
— I hope we shall be more mindful of each other — just for her sake
— learning a quicker tenderness from finding her no more —
So many brave — have died, this year — it don't seem lonely, as it did
— before Battle begun —, then too, dear Uncle — many weep — so you
are not alone —
I cant believe it, while I write — that Mira wont come back — I never shall
believe it. 'Twill always seem to me — and more, as months go by — that
she is on a journey, through pleasant lands — I cannot see — but may
— some day — like her —
Uncle Loring, writes that you are not well — I hope you will soon be
better —
Annie, and Will, will need you more — now Mama, is gone —
Loo will make your Home as sweet, as her fingers can —
She is mine, you know, but I will lend her to you, dear Uncle, because you
need her most —
Mother sends much love — and talks tearfully of you —
        Affy, Emily.

Dickinson's mention of the war served as an indirect reminder to Joel that
in that spring of 1862 his friends at Amherst were still mourning the recent loss
of the village's favorite son, Frazar Stearns, killed at the Battle of New Bern in
mid-March. In addition, Emily's permissive gesture at the letter's end of "loan-
ing" her beloved cousin Lou Norcross to aid the bereft Joel Norcross household
is a fine example of what biographer Richard Sewall calls Dickinson's trait of
"playing Deity." Joel would hear the echo of the familiar line from Revelation,
"I Jesus have sent mine angel."

That the poet employed so many comforts in soothing her uncle suggests
that, by the 1860s, she may have reached full power in her mastery of the consolatory form as she initially conceived it. After 1874, when raw experience reforged
her response to life's ultimate trauma, such letters take on a more immediate
tone and a new focus. Gone are the reassuring contexts, rehearsed dramas, and
set rituals of grief. In their place are starkly personal, even startling, revelations
of the poet's awe at the mystery of death, her concern with immortality replac-

ing thoughts once centered on solacing mortal loss, for Edward Dickinson's absence still stunned his daughter two years after his death. "I dream about father every night, always a different dream," she confessed, "and forget what I am doing daytimes, wondering where he is. Without any body, I keep thinking. What kind can that be?" (L471).

Perhaps no letter she wrote better conveys her struggle for control, her reach for art to aid in coping with death, than the message sent to her sister-in-law Susan Gilbert Dickinson after the loss of Sue and Austin's eight-year-old son Gilbert from typhoid fever in early October of 1883 (L868). A cruel, punishing blow to the Dickinson family, Gib's death prostrated his Aunt Emily, who yet reached out of her own grief to be the consoler. Several fractured attempts at poetry in the middle of her letter finally resolve into a completed quatrain at its close.

> Dear Sue —
> The Vision of Immortal Life has been fulfilled —
> How simply at the last the Fathom comes! The Passenger and not the Sea,
> we find surprises us —
> Gilbert rejoiced in Secrets —
> His Life was panting with them — With what menace of Light he cried
> "Dont tell, Aunt Emily"! Now my ascended Playmate must instruct *me*.
> Show us, prattling Preceptor, but the way to thee!
> He knew no niggard moment — His life was full of Boon — The Playthings
> of the Dervish were not so wild as his —
> No crescent was this Creature — He traveled from the Full —
> Such soar, but never set —
> I see him in the Star, and meet his sweet velocity in everything that flies
> — His Life was like the Bugle, which winds itself away, his Elegy an echo
> — his Requiem ecstasy —
> Dawn and Meridian in one.
> Wherefore would he wait, wronged only of Night, which he left for us —
> Without a speculation, our little Ajax spans the whole —
>> Pass to thy Rendezvous of Light,
>> Pangless except for us —
>> Who slowly ford the Mystery
>> Which thou hast leaped across!
>>> Emily.

Lying on her sickbed, a victim of nervous prostration, the poet understood and, prismlike, refracted to Sue an image of the dear child's brief, unfinished life as an elemental part of God's mystery—a mystery equal in enigma, in surprise, to immortality itself, and, like seas and stars and suns, emblematic of its certainty. Dickinson's sophistication had pushed past willingness to die, past birds and angels, past sweet goodnights and reunions in heaven, to a clearer, more complete vision of the soul's trajectory from seen to unseen, a vision that dominated her later years and the late consolations. Through closer acquaintance with death, she had accepted its validity, if not its pain. As she assured a grieving friend in her last surviving letter of consolation, penned shortly before her own death in the spring of 1886,

Though the great Waters sleep,
That they are still the Deep,
We cannot doubt,
No vacillating God
Ignited this Abode
To put it out — (J1599/Fr1641)

. . .

My own experience enables me to attest to the power of Emily Dickinson's consolations. Through the separate untimely losses of my parents and three siblings, one of Dickinson's poems has, in each instance, risen to mind to become the "granite" rock that anchored my grief—always a different poem, but always a particular one there to lean on.

NOTES

1. Sermon on the Mount, King James Bible, Matthew 5:15–16. "Neither do men light a candle, and put it under a bushel, but on a candlestick; and it giveth light unto all that are in the house. Let your light so shine before men, that they may see your good works, and glorify your Father which is in heaven."

2. Johnson mistakenly incorporates as the poem's first line the phrase, "Pursuing you in your transitions," which Dickinson intended as part of her letter's prose. This confusion seems to have obscured the poem's meaning for Johnson. Franklin corrects the error in his notes to Fr1664.

3. A lost poem, its source is a 1912 letter from Susan Dickinson to Samuel Bowles the younger, in which Sue quotes it.

4. Of Dr. Gridley, Jennie Hitchcock wrote Ann Fiske that he had died "without any change in his feelings that I know of—Tis a sad thing to die with no hope beyond the tomb." Helen Hunt Jackson Papers, University of Colorado, March 23, 1852. For Bowles, see L551, 567, and 591.

5. Other examples of her post-1874 style are letters 517, 596, 630, 671, 677, 738, and 1036.

6. The undated letter was acquired by the Houghton Library, Harvard University, in 1988 from a descendent of Joel Norcross and is housed among the Dickinson Family Papers. Also published in the *Emily Dickinson International Society Bulletin* 7.1 (1995): 2–3. Reprinted by permission of The Houghton Library, Harvard University MS Am 1118.7 © The President and Fellows of Harvard College.

Emily Dickinson is the magical poet for the ages. She is supreme!

I find in Dickinson a life that's truly unique and fascinating. I read the poems over and over from time to time, and I'm always thunderstruck! There's no other word. I'm thunderstruck! I'm riveted right to the ground. Because it's such an unusual voice done with such simplicity, such power. There's a very delicate quality, but then there's a fierceness and a very potent strength. Every aspect [of Dickinson] comes down to a snowflake. "There's a certain Slant of light, / Winter Afternoons — / That oppresses, like the Heft / Of Cathedral Tunes / Heavenly Hurt, it gives us." It just knocks you out! As Charles Nelson Reilly would say, "It's gangbusters!" "Heavenly Hurt, it gives us — / We can find no scar, / But internal difference, Where the Meanings, are." It just echoes. It shakes! It's so powerful. Suddenly you know why you're alive. What it is to be alive. It's to *feel*. To *sense*. Wonderful!

JULIE HARRIS, ACTOR

Excerpted from a 1991 interview by Georgiana Strickland, editor of the *Emily Dickinson International Society Bulletin*, about Harris's role as Emily in William Luce's *The Belle of Amherst*. Reprinted with permission.

From the Province of the Saved
Emily Dickinson and Healing

GREGORY ORR

The voice of the solitary that makes others less alone . . .

STANLEY KUNITZ

More of Emily Dickinson's poems begin with "I" than with any other term. Paradoxically, in lyric, the pronoun of self functions inclusively rather than exclusively. The reader is invited to identify with the poem's speaker for the brief, intensified moment of the poem's unfolding. Although in most poems this lyric invitation is implicit, Whitman states it outright and with typical confidence in the opening lines of "Song of Myself," recognizing that all the deeper emotional and spiritual transactions of his sequence derive from it:

I celebrate myself, and sing myself,
And what I assume, you shall assume
For every atom belonging to me as good belongs to you.

And seventy years after Whitman, William Carlos Williams even more boldly reminds his readers that the journey of the lyric "I" is one in which two travel together: "In the imagination, we are from henceforth (as long as you read) locked in a fraternal embrace, the classic caress of author and reader. We are one. Whenever I say 'I' I mean also 'you.' And so, together, as one, we shall begin."[1]

It may be odd to think of Emily Dickinson, one of our premiere *isolatos*, extending such an intimate invitation. But hasn't she herself both claimed and generalized that pronoun when, in that dance of revelation and evasion that marks her early correspondence with friend and mentor Thomas Wentworth

All citations of Dickinson's poems used in this chapter are from *The Poems of Emily Dickinson*, ed. R. W. Franklin, 3 vols. (Cambridge, Mass.: Harvard Univ. Press, 1998).

Higginson, she notes, "When I state myself, as the Representative of the Verse — it does not mean — me — but a supposed person" (L268)? And is she not also our greatest lyric poet, who, as Keats urged, proved her truths on her own pulse? Proven and tested for authenticity there, in the forge and hothouse of her own passions, these truths become "assumable" (to use Whitman's intriguing word) by readers, who give themselves over to her powerful experiences for the brief moment of the poem, who "become" her. But these same readers, drawn perhaps by curiosity, will need courage as well—Dickinson's invitation is frequently also a challenge: "Dare you see a Soul *at the White Heat?*" (J365/Fr401). In accepting her dare, we must accept risk also; we must approach that place from which her words give off their furious heat—"Then crouch within the door." And we recognize that this image of a narrow furnace door describes the shape of the page, while the soul at white heat is an image for her words burning in a black, fractured fire on the page, casting off darkly luminous sparks.

. . .

In order for a poem to come into being, the poet has had to make herself vulnerable to disorder, has had to approach her threshold, that place where disorder and order meet. This counterintuitive decision to seek disorder, to open oneself to that disorder, is the mark of the lyric poet. It's hidden in Frost's wise insistence: "No tears in the writer, no tears in the reader. No surprise for the writer, no surprise for the reader." It's lyric wisdom to cast off armor, to intuit that you will become stronger by taking in the disorder, opening yourself to it and then mastering it with imagination and the primal ordering powers of poetry.

Do poets really have such extraordinary faith in the power of patterned words? Let's take testimony from Emily Dickinson on this.

> I reckon — when I count at all —
> First — Poets — Then the Sun —
> Then Summer — Then the Heaven of God —
> And then — the List is done —
>
> But, looking back — the First so seems
> To Comprehend the Whole —
> The Others look a needless Show —
> So I write — Poets — All —(J569/Fr533)

To poets or to those who write or read poetry to survive, poetry is "All." Why? Because it allows them to create a symbolic, linguistic model of a volatile subjectivity, be it suffering or joy, not with the aim of abolishing it but of dramatizing it and giving it shape. And by doing this, they will have transformed themselves from passive victim to active, ordering agent. Mind you, it's not a simplistic ordering, not simply a question of transforming chaos into prim cosmos—as if a maelstrom were tamed to become insipid tea in a cup. The poem that results is a dynamic representation of an unfolding interplay of disorder and order, both formal and thematic. Nor is the personal lyric about definitive ordering; it is, in Frost's formula, "a momentary stay against confusion." The efficacy of the lyric must be constantly renewed—new poems must be written as new joys and despairs assert themselves.

Many of Dickinson's greatest poems are tiny dramas of survival, and Dickinson herself is a survivor, one of "the Saved." The writing of her poems is *how* she survived. We, her readers, can also participate in this vitalizing survival by reading her poems. When we read her poems with lyric identification, they enter deeply into us and *her* survival becomes *our* survival; *her* mastery of traumatic experience, *her* triumphant reuniting of feeling and event, becomes *our* triumph. This is the intimate rescue mode of the personal lyric: one self at a time. And only through feeling, through the vulnerability of letting our defenses down and "becoming" Emily, becoming the self of her poems as it undergoes suffering and ecstasy and survives, can we be rescued.

Emily Dickinson knew all this. It's in her poems, this understanding of how poets who have suffered and survived (and voiced their survival) can help other people.

The Province of the Saved
Should be the Art — To save —
Through Skill obtained in Themselves —
The Science of the Grave

No Man can understand
But He that has endured
The Dissolution — in Himself —
That Man — be qualified

To qualify Despair
To Those who failing new —
Mistake Defeat for Death — Each time —
Till acclimated — to — (J539/Fr659)

Forgive my necessarily reductive paraphrase as I tease out one central thread from the poem: poets/people who have survived should take upon themselves the task of helping others survive. These poets have learned the skill/art through their own difficult experiences. No one who hasn't undergone it can understand suffering. Such a person is "qualified" to "qualify" (mitigate) suffering for those to whom it's a new experience, and who, because of their naïveté, think that suffering is death and cannot be survived. Such newcomers to suffering will continue in their mistaken, consecutive despairs, again and again, until they are acclimated to it. Again, forgive the painful clunkiness of this reductive paraphrase, but here's the point—those who suffer and survive (the Saved) have the power and the moral obligation to help others who are new to the process.

To me, this poem describes the poet who has suffered trauma, found "salvation" in writing, and then recognized her calling as the writing of poems, the giving of testimony that will help others to cope with trauma. She and her poems are proof that people can survive extreme physical and psychological states. Her poems help the sufferer to make the crucial distinction between suffering as setback and suffering as utter annihilation. Dickinson may claim, as she does in a letter of consolation to a bereaved friend, Mrs. J. G. Holland, that "there are depths in every Consciousness, from which we cannot rescue ourselves — to which none can go with us — which represent to us Mortally — the Adventure of Death" (L555), but in fact, many of her poems do just that: they accompany us to depths within us that we could not bear alone, and they invite us to ascend to heights with her, through her poems, that we could not dare alone.

· · ·

It's time, of course, to test the theory in its enactments, to encounter those poems in which Dickinson coped with the volatile emotional life that she experienced by turning it into language and shaping it into poems. But it's difficult to decide what thread to follow into the labyrinthine richness of her work. Her volume of collected poems consists of more than seventeen hundred lyrics. Such plenitude can baffle. Between the covers of that thick book, she sounds an astounding variety of notes on the scale of lyric subjectivity: high and low, ecstasy and despair, joy and terror, incoherence and crystalline lucidity. But we must begin somewhere, so why not take survival at its psychic extremity—the self in its most difficult encounter with destructive violence, what we now call trauma. Originally a Greek word for "wound," "trauma" is now used to describe a category of dire experience that threatens to shatter or overwhelm entirely the self's integrity. It is associated with sudden, violent experiences in which the self feels (and often is) utterly powerless. We have also begun to notice (by way of studies of soldiers after combat and women after rape) that the effects of traumatic violence can be ongoing, that it alters the chemistry and functioning of the brain in ways that can permanently undermine the individual from within.

Among her numerous other distinctions, Dickinson is our premiere poet of the traumatic. Her image for trauma? Lightning.

It struck me — every Day —
The Lightning was as new
As if the Cloud that instant slit
And let the Fire through —

It burned Me — in the Night —
It Blistered to My Dream —
It sickened fresh upon my sight —
With every Morn that came —

I thought that Storm — was brief —
The Maddest — quickest by —
But Nature lost the Date of This —
And left it in the Sky — (J362/Fr636)

Hard, important information, testimony to us: for some unfortunates, trauma is not one finished incident but a persistent one that replays itself with excruciating intensity, haunts dreams ("burned me — in the Night — / It Blistered to My Dream"), and continues throughout the day. The poem ends where it began, in a sense, with the stunned wonder that something so intense could also be so long lasting in its harmful effects. But again, as with all lyrics, the poet survived; this poem comes to us from "the Province of the Saved" and brings news that a self can feel this intensely and still stay lucid. This brings us to another great poem of trauma.

The first Day's Night had come —
And grateful that a thing
So terrible — had been endured —
I told my Soul to sing —

She said her Strings were snapt —
Her Bow — to Atoms blown —
And so to mend her — gave me work
Until another Morn —

And then — a Day as huge
As Yesterdays in pairs,
Unrolled its horror in my face —
Until it blocked my eyes —

My Brain — begun to laugh —
I mumbled — like a fool —
And tho' 'tis Years ago — that Day —
My brain keeps giggling — still.

And Something's odd — within —
That person that I was —
And this One — do not feel the same —
Could it be Madness — this? (J410/Fr423)

We don't know what happened on that first day because Dickinson's poems are always more existential essence than circumstantial detail. But it could well have been a single lightning bolt of trauma—certainly it shattered the soul's harp and no immediately consoling song could be sung. And yet, to repair that harp both self and soul were kept busy through the long, sleepless night that follows such days. But what the next dawn brought was worse, was somehow a doubled horror in the face of which the self lost utterly its precarious stability. It's only then, as late as line 11, that we learn that the instigating first night took place years ago. But its impact on the consciousness, on the mind itself, produced a persistent form of hysterical laughter—a deeply inappropriate response to horror (colored, a bit, by the gothic image of a madman)—which is followed by three lines of lucid testimony about an altered self: "Something's odd — within — / That person that I was — / And this One — do not feel the same." Her rhetorical question in the final line is, of course, warranted by the awfulness of what she's endured and how it has altered her. Warranted as long as we can (and we do) respond to the question with a resounding no. No, this isn't madness—because you understood and remembered everything and because you did not passively endure your experience but turned it into words and shaped it into this passionate articulation of suffering. No, this isn't madness, because you survived and wrote this and we readers who might also have suffered something that felt like what you describe—we cannot help but take courage from how you have survived and clearly triumphed.

Maybe she didn't succumb to madness, but certainly she knows that, with a sensibility as intense and volatile as hers, it's a real possibility. And so, she writes that poem also, a poem of intimate catastrophe. What courage!—the self un-folding the narrative of its own extinction through a despair or inner collapse.

I felt a Funeral, in my Brain,
And Mourners to and fro
Kept treading — treading — till it seemed
That Sense was breaking through —

And when they all were seated,
A Service, like a Drum —
Kept beating — beating — till I thought
My Mind was going numb —

And then I heard them lift a Box
And creak across my Soul
With those same Boots of Lead, again,
Then Space — began to toll,

As all the Heavens were a Bell,
And Being, but an Ear,
And I, and Silence, some strange Race
Wrecked, solitary, here —

And then a Plank in Reason, broke,
And I dropped down, and down —
And hit a World, at every plunge,
And Finished knowing — then — (J280/Fr340)

And yet, of course, for all the vividness and authenticity of the above poem, she did not "finish knowing then." She survived and persisted. Which is not to say that she did not suffer for each of these poems, did not earn them through enduring them in her hours of solitude.

Supreme poet of anguished consciousness that she is, Dickinson knows that the dangers within the self, the self-hauntings, are far more frightening than anything one might meet in the natural or even supernatural world.

One need not be a Chamber — to be Haunted —
One need not be a House —

The Brain has Corridors — surpassing
Material Place —

Far safer, of a Midnight Meeting
External Ghost
Than its interior Confronting —
That Cooler Host.

Far safer, through an Abbey gallop,
The Stones a'chase —
Than Unarmed, one's a'self encounter —
In lonesome Place —

Ourself behind ourself, concealed —
Should startle most. . . . (J670/Fr407)

How much we learn about the perils of being from her work. When I read the lines

After great pain — a formal feeling comes
The Nerves sit ceremonious, like Tombs —

I don't feel I am hearing about her interest in meter but about that aspect of trauma that results in numbness.

The still Heart questions was it He, that bore,
And Yesterday, or Centuries before?

The Feet, mechanical, go round —
Of Ground, or Air, or Ought —
A Wooden way
Regardless grown,
A Quartz contentment, like a stone —

This is the Hour of Lead —
Remembered, if outlived,
As Freezing persons, recollect the Snow —
First — Chill — then Stupor — then the letting go — (J341/Fr372)

And surely numbness after trauma—to survive the experience, but only at the price of having lost the ability to feel—is one of the great perils of being human.

Dickinson also writes about how trauma can restrict the range of our subsequent emotional lives by acclimating us to negative feelings but unfitting us for those at the positive end of the spectrum.

> I can wade Grief —
> Whole Pools of it —
> I'm used to that —
> But the least push of Joy
> Breaks up my feet —
> And I tip — drunken . . . (J252/Fr312)

She can hymn desolation and agony.

> The Heart asks Pleasure — first —
> And then — Excuse from Pain —
> And then — those little Anodynes
> That deaden suffering —
>
> And then — to go to sleep —
> And then — if it should be
> The will of its Inquisitor
> The privilege to die — (J536/Fr588)

She can endure and dramatize the impact of wrenching loss.

> Empty my Heart, of Thee —
> Its single Artery —
> Begin, and leave Thee out —
> Simply Extinction's Date —
>
> Much Billow hath the Sea —
> One Baltic — They —
> Subtract Thyself, in play,
> And not enough of me
> Is left — to put away —
> "Myself" meant Thee —

Erase the Root — no Tree —
Thee — then — no me —
The Heavens stripped —
Eternity's vast pocket, picked — (J587/Fr393)

She shrewdly rehearses the ways in which we try to adjust to agony.

It don't sound so terrible — quite — as it did —
I run it over — "Dead," Brain, "Dead."
Put it in Latin — left of my school —
Seems it don't shriek so — under rule.

Turn it, a little — full in the face
A Trouble looks bitterest —
Shift it — just —
Say "When Tomorrow comes this way —
I shall have waded down one Day." . . . (J426/Fr384)

She faces the loss of a beloved with courage and without undue reliance on the otherworldly consolations that conventional Christianity makes available, preferring instead the spirited attachments to this world symbolized by the primer.

Not in the World to see his face —
Sounds long — until I read the place
Where this — is said to be
But just the Primer — to a life
Unopened — rare — Upon the Shelf —
Clasped yet — to Him — and me —

And yet — My Primer suits me so
I would not choose — a Book to know
Than that — be sweeter wise —
Might some one else — so learned — be —
And leave me — just my A — B — C —
Himself — could have the Skies — (J418/Fr435)

Grief and loss take her over and force her into song, but she is too strong to yield to these agonies. Nor will she permit her enormously complex subjective life to be restrained in any way, especially by those who wish to keep her still and shut her up by restricting her access to poetry, by (God forbid) limiting her to the clumsy stumble of prose.

> They shut me up in Prose —
> As when a little Girl
> They put me in the Closet —
> Because they like me "still" —
>
> Still! Could themself have peeped —
> And seen my Brain — go round —
> They might as wise have lodged a Bird
> For Treason — in the Pound —
>
> Himself has but to will
> And easy as a Star
> Abolish his Captivity —
> And laugh — No more have I — (J613/Fr445)

Such defiant exuberance with which this poem ends! Dickinson knows the dull stabilities of narrative and prose are not for her—not true to the wildness of her spirit and imagination. She will not be tamed. Or will she? Who can find the end to the mysteries of our humanness?

> Not with a Club, the Heart is broken
> Nor with a Stone —
> A Whip so small you could not see it
> I've known
>
> To lash the Magic Creature . . . (J1304/Fr1349)

Aware of what is perpetually at stake existentially, she has sobering advice for those who might wish to remain graceful and aesthetic in their suffering.

> Floss wont save you from an Abyss,
> But a Rope will —
> Notwithstanding a Rope for a Souvenir
> Is not beautiful —

But I tell you every step is a Trough —
And every stop a Well —
Now will you have the Rope or the Floss?
Prices reasonable — (J1322/Fr1335)

She can articulate a sense of cryptic wonder.

I am afraid to own a Body —
I am afraid to own a Soul —
Profound — precarious Property . . . (J1090/Fr1050)

Or she can brood on the loss of religious faith and the certainties it gave.

Those — dying then,
Knew where they went —
They went to God's Right Hand —
That Hand is amputated now
And God cannot be found. . . . (J1551/Fr1581)

But she can also hymn the destabilizings of ecstasy in a poem which I take as an incantatory, erotic paean by someone who may or may not have known intimate sexuality but certainly imagined a vivid and idealized version of its satisfactions.

Wild Nights — Wild Nights!
Were I with thee
Wild Nights would be
Our luxury!

Futile — the Winds —
To a Heart in port —
Done with the Compass —
Done with the Chart!

Rowing in Eden —
Ah, the Sea!
Might I but moor — Tonight —
In Thee! (J249/Fr269)

And her poem of gratitude to Higginson for his interest in her work shows her passion in its most affirmative mode.

> As if I asked a common Alms,
> And in my wondering hand
> A Stranger pressed a Kingdom,
> And I, bewildered, stand —
> As if I asked the Orient
> Had it for me a Morn —
> And it should lift its purple Dikes,
> And shatter me with Dawn! (J323/Fr14)

. . .

Having touched lightly on the infinitely intense and various nature of Dickinson's subjectivity, I want to pause to stress a particular aspect of stabilization in her work. Having asserted that the personal lyric is a superbly designed instrument for processing the experience of disorder, I still have to marvel at Dickinson's achievement and her survival. How does she endure such repeated, intense vulnerability to experience? No—how does she survive it *and* succeed in expressing and shaping it without being overwhelmed?

We can note that she does not invent new thematic ideas for ordering her subjectivity as, say, both Wordsworth and Whitman had. She is not a visionary reorderer of consciousness in that sense. Nor did she develop and deploy, as Whitman did, new formal principles in order to express a new way of being in the world. She is closer to Baudelaire, another volatile subjectivity, in her "solution." I think one of the secrets of her success is her reliance on inherited formal structures for her utterances.

It is the certainty of the stability of her forms that allows her to be so free, so uninhibited and bold in their content. This restless, reckless poet needed something she could count on. And she counted on the "numbers" of traditional form. Not for her the bold innovations of the city dwellers. Her boldness is elsewhere than in issues of formal appearance. She will inhabit (with her wildness) what dwellings are already there: variations on the hymn meter that was the most available to her consciousness in that church-saturated, provincial world she inhabited. She took the church meter and used it for secular purposes: to stabilize the self as it dramatizes its vulnerabilities and instabilities, its epiphanies and catastrophes.

How much stability must have been granted her at the outset of her poems, knowing they would most often unfold as a given form. But no sooner do we recognize traditional form in her work than we immediately notice what she does with the forms, to the forms. Dickinson is such a lively and indelible personality, possessed of (and by) such a powerful linguistic imagination that she cannot help but warp these frail meters into something strikingly free and eccentric like herself. When I think of how Dickinson distorted her inherited forms and tangled their syntax with her passion, I think of Coleridge's epigram about another great transformer of forms, John Donne.

> With Donne, whose muse on dromedary trots,
> Wreathe iron pokers into true-love knots;
> Rhyme's sturdy cripple, fancy's maze and clue,
> Wit's forge and fire-blast, meaning's press and screw.

Not only could this epigram apply equally (as if *avant la lettre*) to Dickinson, but it even uses images of intensity ("forge" and "fire-blast"; the torture instruments of "press and screw") that she herself used in poems.

> Essential Oils — are wrung —
> The Attar from the Rose
> Be not expressed by Suns — alone —
> It is the gift of Screws. . . . (J675/Fr772)

Yes, this is a poem about perfume, but it's also about lyric poetry and her process of making it.

More or less unconcerned about form (if one can say this of a great artist), Dickinson was free to take on the primary task of ordering her enormous verbal and imaginative energy and her emotional chaos into vivid articulation. Her meeting of subjectivity with form is a far happier event than, say, that of Wordsworth with the sonnet form. Wordsworth, by and large, retreated into form as his imaginative power and emotional courage faded in midlife. The sonnet's narrowness (he compared it to a nun's cell) was more than enough room for his diminished, diminishing self. Not so with Dickinson and form: she was always bursting it or mocking its expectations with her off-rhymes or complete abandonment of rhyme, her casual attitude toward meter. The iambic norm bores her or fails to suit the intensity of intellect and emotion she brings to her poems. She must strain and distort her rhythms. And as for syntax, that fundamental guide to meaning, be brave as you approach a Dickinson poem; arm yourself with patience before you try to unknot its intricacies. She warns us herself that neatness is not her forte: "When I try to organize — my little Force explodes — and leaves me bare and charred" (L271).

And yet, she knew exactly what she was up to, knew she both needed form and was not form's slave. When her epistolary mentor, Thomas Higginson, responded to her second batch of poems by noting that her poems had only an ungainly grip on conventional prosody, she put him neatly in his place: "you think my gait 'spasmodic' — I am in danger — Sir" (L265). What a glorious retort! "I am in danger, sir," she says, mimicking a helpless Victorian heroine who addresses her plaintive appeal to a male hero. As if she needed his help to smooth her lines; as if she didn't know what she was doing and with utmost, powerful intent. To be fair to Higginson (whom I admire for his care of her, his respect for her), he recognized very quickly in their relationship that she was a genius and that his function really was just to say to her, You are not alone and without intelligent readers—I know how good you are (though I am afraid to introduce you to the world, because you are so strange and powerful and will not fit the patronizing definitions we have for female poets).

And to be further fair to Dickinson, her gait was spasmodic, as well it might be in order to accurately dramatize her sense of existential jeopardy.

I stepped from Plank to Plank
A slow and cautious way
The Stars about my Head I felt
About my Feet the Sea.

I knew not but the next
Would be my final inch —
This gave me that precarious Gait
Some call Experience. (J875/Fr926)

Dickinson's distortions and warping of form include also her punctuation. Although her dashes are clearly a product of her genius—dramatically effective expressive distortions—they can also seem willfully bizarre and interfere with a poem's meaning, especially for beginning and intermediate readers. Her eccentric punctuation put me off and puzzled me for decades. What I've ended up doing, in order to continually deepen my love and appreciation for her work, is to try to put the punctuation aside and read a poem of hers aloud, searching out the appropriate pauses and the tone of voice that could be saying those particular words, doing my best to find the person speaking her way through the syntactic twists and hesitations, the associative leaps and oracular abruptness of these strange poems.

And doing so, becoming her by saying her words aloud, how much I gain. How her poems enrich me with their extraordinary emotional range. She seems to me the equal of Shakespeare, though in a lyric mode. He created a hundred vivid characters moving through the world; she dramatized several hundred vivid emotional states in the course of her work. It's not that she showed us that her inner world of subjectivity (and ours, by analogy) was rich and complex (we knew that), but that she showed us it could be given voice and form. Keats, wishing near the end of his life not only to write poems but to "do some good," had come around to a grudging admiration of Wordsworth because he "thinks into the human heart." He even posited, in a wonderful image, that poets like Wordsworth, feeling "the Burden of the Mystery," were writing poems that were "explorative of the dark passages," and it's clear from his image that these dark passages are corridors in the human mind, aspects of consciousness itself. Keats wrote to his friend that, if they both lived long enough, they, too, might engage in such an exploration, to the benefit of mankind. Of course, Keats didn't live long enough, but Dickinson did. It's possible to think of her as exploring, with the huge body of her poems, more dark passages than anyone before or since in English. She's like a great inner spelunker—her own mind and subjectivity a veritable Carlsbad Caverns of tunnels and chambers and strange spaces full of wonder and mystery and terror.

I don't think anyone can or should tell another person what poems of Dickinson's are the ones to go to. She is a long valley we each have to walk on our own. I don't even necessarily think that whole poems are essential. Sometimes a mere line or two of hers has in it the wisdom and healing that is all I need to restore myself or to recognize myself—and that's not an easy confession for me to make, since I'm a lyric poet myself, and we poets are pledged to the dogma that each poem is sacred in its entirety. But why should that be? Dickinson was clearly oracular, epigrammatic, pithy—why shouldn't we derive insight, consolation, or revelation from isolated passages as well as whole poems?

In so many of her poems, even the oddest, I feel as if she's telling me, telling us, Don't be afraid to be human, to be passionate and strange to the fullest extent of your being, to be yourself completely. And listening to her, reading her poems aloud, I become her briefly when her feelings and mine coincide, and when that happens I feel her coaxing me with her own example toward an amazing bravery.

NOTE

1. William Carlos Williams, *Spring and All (1923)*. *Imaginations* (New York: New Direction Books, 1970), 178.

"There came a Day at Summer's full —"

Ellen Bacon

The death of my husband, composer Ernst Bacon, on the morning of March 16, 1990, was not unexpected. At two months short of ninety-two years, he had lived a long, full, rich life. Besides having congestive heart failure, he had struggled for thirteen years with diminishing sight in his one remaining eye, having lost the other in an unsuccessful operation.

After meeting with family members at the hospital that morning, I spent the rest of the day phoning Ernst's distant relatives and old friends around the country. By evening I was exhausted and knew that the time had come to face my aloneness in the empty house. Instinctively I was drawn to Ernie's study in the basement, where he had spent so many hours for so many years, absorbed in composing music.

Ernst was best known for his many song settings of Emily Dickinson's poetry, composed between the late 1920s and the late 1960s. As far as I knew, he had not written anything in this genre during our marriage; but as I entered the study that night, my eye fell immediately on a manuscript setting of "There came a day at summer's full."

There came a day at summer's full,
Entirely for me;
I thought that such were for the saints,
Where revelations be.

The sun, as common, went abroad,
The flowers, accustomed, blew,
As if no sail the solstice passed
That maketh all things new.

All citations of Dickinson's poems used in this chapter are from *The Poems of Emily Dickinson,* ed. Martha Dickinson Bianchi and Alfred Leete Hampson (Boston: Little, Brown, 1936).

The time was scarce profaned by speech;
The symbol of a word
Was needless, as at sacrament
The wardrobe of our Lord.

Each was to each the sealèd church,
Permitted to commune this time,
Lest we too awkward show
At supper of the Lamb.

The hours slid fast, as hours will,
Clutched tight by greedy hands;
So faces on two decks look back,
Bound to opposing lands.

And so, when all the time had failed,
Without external sound,
Each bound the other's crucifix,
We gave no other bond.

Sufficient troth that we shall rise —
Deposed, at length, the grave —
To that new marriage, justified
Through Calvaries of Love! (J322/Fr325)

Reading these words, previously unknown to me, I was overwhelmed by both grief and joy—grief in feeling the full impact of my loss, and joy in realizing that the bond of love could continue beyond the grave. Not only did I feel profoundly comforted by Dickinson's words, pointing to a resurrection of marriage on a spiritual level, but also deeply relieved that Ernst, who had been essentially an agnostic, must have wanted to believe this too.

This poem not only enabled me to confront fully the sorrow of the moment but also gave me courage to cope with the coming days of bereavement. Although a great many of Emily Dickinson's poems have been meaningful in my life, I will always be especially grateful for "There came a day at summer's full," which opened an important spiritual vista when I needed it most.

In later weeks, I found another song in Ernie's study, clearly the last of his sixty-seven Dickinson settings. On the super-enlarged staff paper that he needed in his near blindness was his handwritten setting of "I died for beauty." I'm sure he knew that his time on earth was coming to a close, and Emily's words must have reassured him that he had fulfilled the purpose of his life—to express his own truth and beauty in his writing and compositions.

> I died for beauty, but was scarce
> Adjusted in the tomb,
> When one who died for truth was lain
> In an adjoining room.
>
> He questioned softly why I failed?
> "For beauty," I replied.
> "And I for truth, — the two are one;
> We brethren are," he said.
>
> And so, as kinsmen met a night,
> We talked between the rooms,
> Until the moss had reached our lips,
> And covered up our names. (J449/Fr448)

As it turned out, "I died for beauty" must have been the only Dickinson poem that Ernst set to music during the time that we were married. Upon later scrutiny, I realized that the manuscript of "There came a day" was not a recent work, as I had first thought, but the original of an already published version. I now believe that he composed this setting to console himself after the death of his previous wife and purposely left it on top of his desk for me to find after his own death. No gift could have been a greater blessing and balm, and both manuscripts will always be special treasures to me.

For about three years after Ernie's death, I often had dreams in which he was still with me, dreams that were so real that when I awakened in the morning, I was truly confused as to whether or not he had actually died. These dreams finally came to an end, but in my waking hours I still feel his support and encouragement in countless ways and am constantly influenced by his viewpoints, from the mundane to the sublime.

Our "new marriage" has sustained me through the years, as has his music and, through his songs, Emily Dickinson's poetry. The words and music of one song, in particular, come to me almost daily when I walk the dogs in the last light of the day.

The Sun went down —
No man looked on,
The Earth and I alone
Were present at the majesty;
He triumphed and went on.

The Sun went up —
No man looked on,
The Earth and I and One —
A nameless bird, a stranger,
Were witness for the Crown. (J1079/Fr1109)

Walking into the setting sun on the Erie Canal towpath, time and again I've felt that Ernie was there with me, "present at the majesty," "witness for the Crown"—and I'm always grateful for his companionship and for the poet who gave him the words to express his deepest, most enduring emotions.

It's true about her consolatory power, and I've noticed that many people who don't read much poetry are devoted to her, doubtless in part for that reason. Aside from the substance of her poems, I also think she invites people to commune with her by the homemade feeling of her poems and their use of hymn meters. Brilliant as she is, there is a Down Home flavor to her work, and it doesn't come on as Art.

RICHARD WILBUR, POET

"This Consciousness that is aware"
The Consolation of Emily Dickinson's Phenomenology

JOY LADIN

This Consciousness that is aware
Of Neighbors and the Sun
Will be the one aware of Death ... (J822/Fr817)

Some years ago, I taught a community education seminar at the Emily Dickinson Homestead called "Of Consciousness, her awful Mate" that focused exclusively on Dickinson's phenomenological poems—that is, the poems in which Dickinson attempts to describe the anatomy of consciousness. These poems have always appealed to me as metaphysical contortionist acts, efforts to use language to enable the soul to see what it looks like with its eyes closed. But the subject soon lost its theoretical cast when one of the participants, an octogenarian, reported that her husband had died shortly after the first meeting. She herself was so frail it was hard to imagine how she could bear the weight of her loss. I suggested, with what I hoped was tact, that perhaps she didn't feel up to coming to class. But she insisted on attending. She and her husband had been reading the poems I'd assigned virtually up to the moment of his death, she told us. Her husband had loved them, and they both had felt that Dickinson's words were easing the incomprehensible transition as his life slipped through their hands.

Even as I welcomed her continued participation, I couldn't help but wonder how Dickinson's poems had helped them. While Dickinson certainly participated in her era's sentiment-soaked approach to death and mourning, in the selection of poems I had assigned, her attitude is detached, almost sardonic. For example, take the first stanza of "A Solemn thing within the Soul" (J483/Fr467), a poem that suspends awareness of mortality between the calipers of phenomenological examination.

All citations of Dickinson's poems used in this chapter are from *The Poems of Emily Dickinson*, ed. R. W. Franklin, 3 vols. (Cambridge, Mass.: Harvard Univ. Press, 1998).

A Solemn thing within the Soul
To feel itself get ripe —
And golden hang — while farther up —
The Maker's Ladders stop —
And in the Orchard far below —
You hear a Being — drop. . . .

The moment of awareness that this poem describes—the "Solemn thing" that is the recognition of one's own mortality—is normally fraught with feeling. Dickinson drains away such subjectivity, offering instead a dispassionate portrayal purged of any characteristics that might identify "the Soul" with one individual or another. Such abstracting, generalizing effects are built into phenomenology. When consciousness becomes the object of its own analytical attention, the reticent, enigmatic recesses we normally think of as our most intimate selves are turned inside out and projected as a featureless psychic model. Dickinson's mappings of this model soul magnify our deepest, most delicate sensations, making them visible to us, enabling us to reflect on and articulate them. But in doing so, they depersonalize those sensations, presenting as categorizable what we normally experience as idiosyncratic gestalts of feeling. In this sense, phenomenological consciousness is indeed an "awful mate" for the soul (J894/Fr1076).

Dickinson never tired of turning the cold eye of phenomenology on intimate states of psychic distress, such as the ripening shudder of mortality. In fact, Dickinson portrays detached self-awareness as a normal, or at least unavoidable, response to anguish, grief, and death. For example, in "After great pain, a formal feeling comes," the observing consciousness circulates like a visitor at a wake: "The Nerves sit ceremonious, like Tombs — / The stiff Heart questions was it He, that bore, / And yesterday, or Centuries before?" (J341/Fr372). Susan Manning has noted that for both Dickinson and her younger but equally phenomenology-besotted contemporary William James, "The continuance of consciousness is . . . a tragic fact in life: because consciousness is characteristically longer lived than the objects of its attention, its experience, unrelentingly, must be of loss."[1] But for Dickinson, phenomenological detachment in the face of "great pain" also represents a sort of triumph, the resistance of consciousness to circumstances that threaten to annihilate it. Like Ishmael at the end of *Moby-Dick*, Dickinson's consciousness is always there to watch the shattered psyche swirl down the drain—or, as she puts it with exquisite phenomenological precision, to register "internal difference, / Where the Meanings, are" (J258/Fr320).

Indeed, for Dickinson, anguish, grief, and even death cannot be separated from the self-regarding spectacle of consciousness.

> This Consciousness that is aware
> Of Neighbors and the Sun
> Will be the one aware of Death
> And that itself alone
>
> Is traversing the interval
> Experience between
> And most profound experiment
> Appointed unto Men —
>
> How adequate unto itself
> Its properties shall be
> Itself unto itself and None
> Shall make discovery.
>
> Adventure most unto itself
> The Soul condemned to be —
> Attended by a single Hound
> Its own identity. (J822/Fr817)

For Dickinson, as this poem suggests, death actually heightens consciousness. Even as the soul traverses this "most profound experiment," consciousness continues to record and reflect, examining death with the scientific detachment that the word "experiment" suggests. Yet death is not the subject of this experiment but only a medium, a sort of acid test that reveals the ultimate adequacy that keeps the soul under its own phenomenological microscope throughout and apparently after the dying process, transforming every throe into an assay of its own properties. Indeed, rather than extinguishing "This Consciousness that is Aware," death demonstrates its ineradicable continuance.

Dickinson often presents this continuance of phenomenological awareness as a tragic fact—the soul is "condemned to be" its own "Adventure," apparently for all eternity. But as the poem's confident tone suggests, this undying self-awareness also represents, in radically secularized terms, the soul's victory over death, its relegation of death to one item among the many of which "Consciousness . . . is aware." For Dickinson, phenomenology *is* consolation—perhaps the only consolation that consciousness can offer or receive in a modern world of faltering faith where "God's Right Hand" is "amputated" and "God cannot be found" (J1551/Fr1581). The poet's insistence, bleak as it is, may have comforted my student and her husband as they watched together over the failing of his senses, their vigil lit by the medical machinery that measures the moment-by-moment "ripening of the soul" in terms of the deterioration of pulse and breath. Dickinson's unsentimental charting of the psychic terrain between the moment the soul "feel[s] itself get ripe" and the moment it "hear[s] . . . Being — drop" offers a consoling image of the independence of consciousness from the tragic gravity of death.

But as "This Consciousness that is aware" and other poems suggest, for Dickinson, the independence afforded by phenomenological detachment does not constitute escape. Like the loneliness that one poem describes as "the Maker of the Soul," Dickinson's phenomenological forays not only open the caverns and corridors of our psyches but plunge us into them (J777/Fr877). We find ourselves wandering among tomblike nerves and fingering the asymmetrical lobes of cleft brains, "golden hanging" on the boughs of the tree that, for Dickinson, bears knowledge not of good and evil—terms that have little meaning in her lexicon—but of life and death.

This approach to phenomenology differs from that of William James and other philosophers and psychologists who treat the soul as an analytical subject that can be objectively examined. For Dickinson, phenomenology is enacted not through objective analysis per se—such as in the "pure phenomenology" of Husserl—but through the unfolding of language.[2] We cannot sit back and peruse Dickinson's maps of the soul; we must complete and enter into them through the act of interpretation. For example, the opening sentence of "This Consciousness that is aware" unwinds over eight lines and two stanzas—fully half the poem. As we make our way from line to line, our sense of that sentence—and thus our sense of this consciousness—keeps shifting. The first line puts consciousness—stripped down to its fundamental quality and activity: awareness—center stage. However, the second line, grammatically a direct extension of the first, shifts our focus to the external objects of consciousness: "Neighbors and the Sun." In the third line, our attention is wrenched from those current objects of awareness to the future object that, it seems, will replace them all: death. However, the fourth line puts death in its place, asserting that death will simply clear the way for the gaze of consciousness to settle on its ultimate object: "itself alone." While the phenomenological twists and turns of the sentence continue for four more lines, the first stanza demonstrates how intimately entwined Dickinson's analysis of the soul is with our process of interpreting the words in which she presents it. Thanks to Dickinson's famous idiosyncrasies of diction, syntax, and punctuation, that process is ongoing; her phenomenology never crystallizes into a stable, paraphrasable form that can be abstracted from her specific language.

Because we cannot get at Dickinson's meaning without participating in creating and revising it, her poems refuse to let us view the soul from the detached, intellectual distance to which other forms of phenomenology invite us. Even as Dickinson lays out the soul for phenomenological analysis, the interpretive processes she engenders subtly but inescapably entwine our consciousness with the consciousness on the dissecting table. For philosophers like James and Husserl, detachment and objectivity are preconditions for valid phenomenological work; messier, intermediate relations between self and soul are obstacles to be overcome, impurities to be purified. Dickinson revels in the entire scale of relations, playing back and forth between detachment and identification like a trombone player working the slide. Take "A Solemn thing within the Soul." The opening lines seem to place us at an extreme phenomenological distance, a sort of metaphenomenology—the phrase "to feel itself" suggests the soul's detached awareness of its own sensation of mortality, while we stand at an even greater remove, watching this model soul watch itself "get ripe." But even as this double distance is established, Dickinson complicates and undercuts it. The moment the soul perceives its own ripening—a moment graphically represented by the dash at the end of the second line—the phrase "and golden hang" transforms the abstract, abstracted, self-examining soul into pendulous fullness, simultaneously "golden" and "hanging"; subject to time and suspended in space, it regards its own ripening not from a transcendent phenomenological distance but as one among innumerable fruits swaying from the boughs of the tree of life under the gaze of "the Maker." As for us, our souls have been tangled up with the terms of the poem from the moment the model soul of the first line became the self-regarding, precariously ripening fruit of the third. Phrases like "feel itself get ripe" only have meaning in relation to our own psychic experience. To make sense of them we must provide referents from our own souls. This implicit identification with the soul becomes explicit in the final lines of the stanza: "And in the Orchard far below — / You hear a Being — drop." This switch from third-person observation to direct second-person address is the poetic equivalent of an actor erasing the conventional "fourth wall" of the theater by turning to include the audience in the scene. But this radical shift in our relation to the world of the poem—our sudden inclusion between its margins—does not shock. Rather, as we read the poem, we rewrite ourselves in its terms, thinking of our awareness of mortality via images of apples and ladders. In effect, Dickinson's phenomenological poems not only describe psychic terrain, they partially create it; as the poem's syntax shifts and shudders, so does our sense of our own souls.

Awareness of this mutually constituting, mutually destabilizing relationship between language and consciousness is integral to Dickinson's phenomenology. Her phenomenological poems simultaneously delineate and extend the limits of language, demonstrating that language can never completely capture consciousness, because consciousness keeps growing and changing in response to the words that describe it. In that sense, the maker's verbal ladders always stop short of their phenomenological target. But by the same token, Dickinson's poems insist that consciousness is always open to language, that no matter how harrowing our experience, where language is, the soul is never completely alone.

I imagine the consolation this poem offered my student and her husband had much to do with its insistence on the omnipresence not only of consciousness but also of language. "This Consciousness that is aware" emphasizes the tendency of consciousness toward self-enclosed isolation: "Adventure most unto itself / The Soul condemned to be." But even as the soul's phenomenological self-absorption threatens to cut it off from "Neighbors and the Sun," the process of translating phenomenology into language dissolves that isolation and restores the soul to the larger context of shared humanity. When phenomenology is embodied in words, and when those words are given meaning by a reader, the solipsistic circularity of any given soul becomes transparent, and each detail of its adventure—including death—becomes knowable, intelligible, shared.

As Dickinson notes in a number of poems, words exhaust themselves rapidly in the corridor between life and death. When death begins to turn the soul that ripens into the being that drops, language seems to lose its connective, intersubjective power. Everything that can be said is said over and over, and meaning leaks away under the weight of the knowledge that what hasn't been said never will be. But when Dickinson's fictional corpses address us, they do so in ordinary conversational tones that suggest that the language-depleting isolation of dying is long behind them: "I heard a fly buzz — when I died" (J465/Fr591); "Because I could not stop for Death / He kindly stopped for me" (J712/Fr479); "My life closed twice before its close" (J1732/Fr1773). As my student's husband's body failed, the couple faced not only the silence of death but the possibility that the words that made up their life together would fail too. But for Dickinson, the power of language to make the innermost workings of one soul visible to another voids death's power to vitiate meaning and strand the living and the dying on opposite sides of an unbridgeable abyss. Phenomenological poems like "A Solemn thing within the Soul" present life and death as neighboring states of being whose porous borders pose no obstacle for either consciousness or language. And wherever there is language, there is also relationship; even Dickinson's most agonizing portrayals of isolation address a presumed reader. In this way, Dickinson's words may have shored up faith in the power of language to keep the intimacy between my student and her husband alive.

Of course, togetherness is not the tenor of Dickinson's phenomenological poems; they cast as cold an eye on life and death as any Yeats could have wished for. But despite the chilly gaze they level at existence, these poems are suffused by a peculiar joie de vivre, a sense of intellectual adventure that is most pronounced when they approach the border between life and death, where my student and her husband read them. In the Puritan version of Genesis that Dickinson inherited, the fruit of knowledge is death. Dickinson, as willfully literal as Milton, insists that the equation works in both directions; that is, in her poems, the fruit of death is knowledge. Sometimes, it seems that Dickinson's craving for the knowledge that she imagines accumulating in the minds and bodies of the dying overwhelms even her grief at their loss. While it is always dangerous to identify Dickinson too closely with the speakers of her poems, Dickinson, like the speaker in "The last Night that She lived," never lets the drama of dying distract her from the phenomenological benefits of death: "We noticed smallest things — / Things overlooked before / By this great light upon our minds / Italicized, as 'twere" (J1100/Fr1100). Death, for Dickinson, casts "great light upon our Minds," which makes it her favorite means of phenomenological illumination.

> The Admirations — and Contempts — of time —
> Show justest — through an Open Tomb —
> The Dying — as it were a Height
> Reorganizes Estimate
> And what We saw not
> We distinguish clear —
> And mostly — see not
> What We saw before —
>
> 'Tis Compound Vision —
> Light — enabling Light —
> The Finite — furnished
> With the Infinite —
> Convex — and Concave Witness —

Back — toward Time —
And forward —
Toward the God of Him — (J906/Fr830)

I suggested above that Dickinson's phenomenology, unlike philosophical phenomenology, cannot be abstracted from the language in which it is phrased.
This isn't true of the first stanza of "The Admirations — and Contempts — of
time." The opening two lines could readily be rewritten as a prose pronounce-
ment on the salutary effects of memento mori: death, here, is not a personal
experience, a matter of individual "ripening," loss, or grief; it is a chastening
corrective to myopic social judgments. As Dickinson's disapproving, didactic
tone suggests, we can (and should) attain this "Reorganize[d] Estimate" pri-
or to dying. The "Open Tomb," then, is a rhetorical device to make a satirical
point, a cognitive crutch for those of us unjustly enthralled by transitory "Admirations — and Contempts."

But with the phrase "The Dying"—the peculiar construction signals that
Dickinson's thought is moving beyond conventional bounds—the perspective
of the poem begins to descend into the not-yet-sealed tomb to think about how
death really affects the way we see life. At first, this imaginative phenomenology
(Dickinson obviously lacked firsthand experience of "The Dying") has little content. The last four lines of the first stanza mark rhetorical time as the brute fact
of dying—the fact that dying entails the inestimable loss implied by "see[ing]
not / What We saw before"—takes on weight in the poet's imagination. As in
many passages in Dickinson, in the second stanza, the breakthrough of imagination is signaled by the breakdown of syntax. The form of this breakthrough is
familiar—as in other poems, Dickinson heaps up parallel metaphoric clauses,
each difficult in itself, each purportedly a synonym for a nominally specified
"it."[3] But there is no other sentence in Dickinson's riddling canon that strains
toward this particular "it," the view attained when existence is regarded simultaneously through the lenses of living and dying, the finite and the infinite.

Is this extraordinary perspective merely an intellectual and verbal construct
that, like the "Open Tomb" of the second line, is irrelevant to the actual experience of loss and death, or does it afford consolation? Death has not yet taught
me. But when I imagine my student and her husband reading this poem, I see
them recognizing in each other the separate lenses of Dickinson's "Compound
Vision," a "Convex — and Concave Witness," as Dickinson puts it, in an image
that concretizes the awful complementarity of death and life. I see them grasping
at the poem's promise that the panorama of "time," so mean and ignoble in the
opening lines, will leap into soul-expanding, four-dimensional focus when their

living and dying minds are brought into conjunction, transforming the sad fact of death into the means by which "The Finite [is] furnished / With the Infinite."

In "The Admiration — and Contempts — of time" Dickinson fuses phenomenology and imagination to reach toward a "Compound Vision" that, by definition, is not a "thing within the Soul" that can be observed or remembered. But Dickinson's greatest phenomenological achievements are rooted not in the conjunction but in the collision of the finite with the infinite. In these poems, "The Dying" is not an imagined future but an agonizing memory—a memory so agonizing, in fact, that it threatens the very categories of back and forward, past and present, death and life.

> Of nearness to her sundered Things
> The Soul has special times —
> When Dimness — looks the Oddity —
> Distinctness — easy — seems —
>
> The Shapes we buried, dwell about,
> Familiar, in the Rooms —
> Untarnished by the Sepulchre,
> The Mouldering Playmate comes —
>
> In just the Jacket that he wore —
> Long buttoned in the Mold
> Since we — old mornings, Children — played —
> Divided — by a world —
>
> The Grave yields back her Robberies —
> The Years, our pilfered Things —
> Bright Knots of Apparitions
> Salute us, with their wings —
>
> As we — it were — that perished —
> Themselves — had just remained till we rejoin them —
> And 'twas they, and not ourself
> That mourned. (J607/Fr337)

At first, "Of nearness to her sundered Things" sounds like any other exercise in Dickinsonian phenomenology. Like "A Solemn thing within the Soul," it begins by focusing our attention on a normally hidden facet of the soul's life cycle, and it does so by distinguishing the soul from "things" that pertain to "her." That distinction enables Dickinson to metaphorically map the soul's private, intermittent perception of mortality onto a physical space in which mortality is a constant and public feature, thus placing the soul's feeling of ripeness into the context of broad, shared cycles of existence. Similarly, in "Of nearness to her sundered Things," the soul/thing distinction enables Dickinson to create a space in which the soul's fleeting, intangible experience of "nearness" to that which time has "sundered" takes on solidity, depth, and duration.

But despite Dickinson's vivid rendering, the space in "A Solemn thing within the Soul" remains clearly metaphorical, a way of bringing sensuous specificity to emotion and internal time. By the second stanza's "Of nearness," the distinction between metaphorical space constructed to magnify the inner workings of a model soul, and the nonmetaphorical space and time outside the margins of the poem, dissolves: the "sundered Things" are "Shapes we buried," and the "Rooms" in which they "dwell about" are not poetic stanzas but the structures in which we live our lives. When we cross the white space between first and second stanzas, the temporal, conceptual, and emotional walls that separate past from present, "Rooms" from "Sepulchres," become so "dim" that "the Mouldering Playmate"—the speaker's, ours, some universal corpse of childhood that refuses to leave any of us behind—hardly pauses to shoulder them aside.[4] The past becomes so phantasmagorically "distinct," the present so "dimmed" by the past, that life and death seem to switch places, as if "'twas they, and not ourself / That mourned." In Dickinson's psychologized version of the Christian Resurrection—that eschatologically "special tim[e]" when "The Grave yields back her Robberies"—death *does* have dominion, for life is paralyzed, all but erased, by the dead's return.

"Of nearness to her sundered Things" doesn't map the soul's "special times" of communion with the "sundered"; with near-performative force it insists that we see ourselves as living with the dead. The dead remain so "distinc[t]," so "Untarnished by the Sepulchre" to which time and memory consign them, so rooted in their "old mornings," that our most fundamental existential bearings founder. We can't distinguish past from present, life from death, for to make such distinctions is to bury, kill, sunder our "Mouldering Playmate[s]" again.[5]

Many writers lament the impermeability of time, the ever-thickening walls it places between us and those we lose. Dickinson knew that time is constantly being shattered, that "The Shapes we buried, dwell about, / Familiar, in the Rooms," that, as she put it in one of her letters to Elizabeth Holland, "'It is finished' can never be said of us" (L555). She knew that the greatest agony of loss is persistence: the persistence of those "Bright Knots of Apparitions" whose "Salute" renders unbearable the persistence of "ourself" (death, like phenomenology, collapses plural and singular) and the world that divides us from them.

When my student and her husband read this poem, did its vision console or sadden? Did they find in Dickinson's words a consoling prophecy of consciousness's triumph over death, or a terrifying premonition of the fact that soon there would be no world that would contain them both? Or is the consolation of Dickinson's phenomenology that by laying bare the fraying intersection where consciousness meets death, we find that consciousness against all odds is "adequate unto itself"—that "Untarnished by the Sepulchre," the soul's "awful Mate" endures, bringing into bright, excruciating conjunction the inimical lenses of death and life, the finite and the infinite?

In memory of Shirley Gladstone, robbed by the grave August 14, 2003

Notes

1. See "How Conscious Could Consciousness Grow? Emily Dickinson and William James," in *Soft Canons: American Women Writers and Masculine Tradition,* ed. Karen L. Kilcup (Iowa City: Univ. of Iowa Press, 1999), 321.

2. Jed Deppman has contrasted Dickinson's phenomenology with Husserl's. See "'I Could Not Have Defined the Change': Rereading Dickinson's Definition Poetry," the *Emily Dickinson Journal* 11.1 (2002): 49–80.

3. Deppman discusses Dickinson's thinking-through-writing processes in some detail in his consideration of her "definition" poems. See Deppman, "Dickinson's Definition Poetry."

4. Actually, Dickinson begins eroding the binary distinctions presumed by normative phenomenology from the opening words, inverting the syntax of the first sentence to make the opening words the distance-eroding phrase "of nearness," and fleshing out the abstract soul by assigning it a feminine pronoun. We never perceive this soul from a distinct distance. We hover close to it, peering over its shoulder into the "nearness" between "her" and what "she" has lost. This is the phenomenological equivalent of what, in fiction, we would call indirect discourse, a mode of description that blends the soul's perspective with that of the observer, intertwining the strands of objectivity and subjectivity that philosophical phenomenology scrupulously pries apart. Rather than offering an objective description of subjective experience, the observer articulates the soul's experience of her "special times" as though looking through "her" eyes. Dickinson's syntactical compression reflects and abets this strategy. The fourth line, for example, doesn't specify who "distinctness—easy—seems" refers to—the observing consciousness or the soul herself.

5. It is hard to think of this psychic night of the living dead as "phenomenology," since there is no apparent distance here between the knower and the known. But for Dickinson, phenomenological detachment was only a baby step toward regions of consciousness and soul that can only be, as she says in "After great pain," "remembered, if outlived, / As Freezing persons, recollect the Snow— / First—Chill—then Stupor—then the letting go." For Dickinson, there is no tourism of trauma, no safe phenomenological distance from which to analyze agony. To truly probe what she calls "the Hour of Lead," we must accept the collapse of the sanitizing, sanity-preserving categories by which we constitute our lives.

"If I can stop one Heart from breaking"

BRUCE BODE

If I were to try to put the essence of religion into one sentence, I might put it this way: religion has to do with seeing the part in the whole and with seeing the whole in the part. It has to do with linking the particular to the universal and with linking the universal to the particular. It has to do with experiencing yourself as part of the creativity of the power of Being and with experiencing the creativity of the power of Being within yourself. This understanding of the essence of the religious enterprise comes right from the word "religion" itself. Our English word derives from the Latin *religio,* and the root word, *lig,* which means to tie or bind or to link. So religion has to do with rebinding, retying, relinking, reconnecting, bringing together again what has been separated and split apart. But in this movement to return to wholeness and to reconnect the particular with the universal, religion sometimes gets into too big a hurry . . . to the point of calling the separation a "fall," a fall into sin. But it is in this separation, recapitulated in each human, that the individual is born, and this is the prerequisite for the religious life. You can't be reunited until you have been separated. And that new unity is quite different from the original unity; for now it is a conscious unity. The New Jerusalem is quite different from the Garden of Paradise.

And yet religion, as commonly understood and practiced, tends to devalue the individual and individuality. There is a sense of individual knowledge and judgment being a theft from the gods, as in the Genesis story—each globe of knowledge plucked from the Tree of Knowledge is experienced as the taking of forbidden fruit so that instead of seeing the enlargement of individual consciousness as part of the growth of the consciousness of God and of Being, religion tends to grind the individual into the dust of the earth along with the tempting serpent.

All citations of Dickinson's poems used in this chapter are from *The Poems of Emily Dickinson,* ed. Thomas H. Johnson, 3 vols. (Cambridge, Mass.: Harvard Univ. Press, 1955).

This was the kind of religious setting in which a bright sensitive young woman from Amherst, Massachusetts, found herself about a century and a half ago. When Emily Dickinson attended Mount Holyoke Female Seminary at age seventeen, revival was in the air. Scholars count at least eight different revivals that swept through Amherst in Emily's formative years. It was the call to give your heart, to commit yourself to greater purity. But something in Emily Dickinson would not allow her to give herself away to the group. According to one story, Dickinson remained seated when, during a revival, those wanting to be Christians were asked to rise. Later, she remarked in a comment to a friend: "They thought it queer I didn't rise; I thought a lie would be queerer."

It's not that she was irreligious but perhaps, in her own way, she took religion even more seriously than others who did rise to the call. Perhaps she believed that her own feelings and thoughts, which were sacred to her, should not be curbed or dissolved into those of the crowd. As Emily Dickinson fought through to her own sense of identity and self-reliance, she came to the conclusion stated in the poem "Much Madness is divinest Sense" (J435/Fr620). And as biographer Richard Sewall suggests, since her private religion took her so far away from orthodox and public religion, she felt that the burden of proof rested on her. And that burden of proof was a mighty one, given her Puritan heritage and her own sensitive nature. You can see and feel the struggle in many of her poems.

Emily Dickinson found her individual soul in her "father's House," as she put it. She lived in her father's house all her life, in the later years not leaving her room or the yard. So her life was in many ways very circumscribed, but she found enough—not only an adequacy but an amplitude. She found not only her individual identity but the connection of that identity to the universal, and she expressed it in the poem "On a Columnar self — / How ample to rely" (J789/Fr740).

Emily Dickinson kept careful track of the various movements of her soul. This was something that those of her Puritan religious heritage were encouraged to do—to keep track of their dealings with God, the power of Being, to ask themselves, What has God wrought in me today? How is God dealing with me today?

She kept track for herself first of all, sometimes sharing her observations in letters with friends. She did not know that she would gain such an audience for her daily diary. We are the blessed recipients of the careful watch she kept of her soul's developments and movements. She cut a deep path into the dark forest of original experience, a path that we may now follow and from which we can make our own small forays into uncharted wilderness areas of interior experience.

If I can draw for a moment on the theological doctrine that was very alive in her day, Emily Dickinson has made a kind of vicarious, or substitutionary, atonement for us. By her strength and willingness to endure suffering, and by her skill in reporting it, she has given to us, without knowing or planning it, the very substance of her life, her very lifeblood, and through her sacrifice, others have been saved, discovered that they are not alone, gained strength, taken heart, and been refreshed.

Although Emily Dickinson struggled with the ultimate questions of existence and the divine level of things, struggled with her faith in the goodness of creation and its power, ultimately she came through and found a way to contribute to the world: to follow your heart, to touch with compassion the lives that come within the scope of your existence. Follow your heart both in terms of its natural sympathetic response to others and the specific contribution that you can make to life. I can imagine the poet asking, "What good am I in the world? My little life is so limited in scope. I can't bring myself to go to church with the others. I can't make myself believe as others believe. I can hardly make it out of my house. My habits are thought to be so odd. But what I can do is 'stop one Heart from breaking' by offering the thoughts, feelings, and words of my poetry and thus 'not live in vain'" (J919/Fr982). The poet's sympathy, compassion, and sense of connection is such that she gives hope for continued relationships even from inside the grave itself.

Note

This essay, in a slightly different form, is excerpted from a four-part sermon series, "Themes from Emily Dickinson," delivered in 2001 by the Reverend Bruce A. Bode. The entire text of this sermon can be viewed at http://www.fountainstreet.org/literature/Sermons-Printed/so6100bode.pdf.

"It ceased to hurt me"

Emily Dickinson's Language of Consolation

CINDY MACKENZIE

The power to console is not within corporeal reach—though its' attempt, is precious.

LETTER 596, EMILY DICKINSON TO MRS. HENRY HILLS

The process of healing "after great pain" can seem interminable, a process that friends and family, sympathetic as they are, cannot truly share or abbreviate. Part of the problem is that we are so completely destabilized by the shock of intense emotional pain that our fractured identity entirely changes our worldview, and with it the way we see all our relationships. We become disassociated. We cannot answer to the ordinary demands of and responsibilities toward others because our energy is so wholly directed toward tending to the pain of the wound within. We become, in a sense, suspended in time, carrying out the necessary routine activities of life yet far more engaged with our inner workings. Our sense of vision seems to change places. We acquire a kind of metaphysical lucidity, sensitively attuned to our inner selves yet reduced to a nebulous, hazy sense of the commonplace realities around us. Nevertheless, we also find that, as much as we try to distract ourselves from the frequent and sometimes constant pangs of inner pain, as much as we resist embarking on the dark and lonely road toward self-healing, in the end we know that we are compelled to turn inward to do the necessary psychological and spiritual work in order to fully enter life again. In eight short lines, Emily Dickinson describes this experience with keen insight.

A Doubt if it be Us
Assists the staggering Mind

All citations of Dickinson's poems used in this chapter are from *The Poems of Emily Dickinson*, ed. R. W. Franklin, 3 vols. (Cambridge, Mass.: Harvard Univ. Press, 1998).

In an extremer Anguish
Until it footing find —

An Unreality is lent,
A merciful Mirage
That makes the living possible
While it suspends the lives. (J859/Fr903)

These were the feelings I had when my marriage ended. Initially, I tried to fill the emptiness I felt with unlikely romantic partners, with indulgences in socializing, with the acquisition of material possessions, with just about anything that would distract me from my painful reality, but I was persistently reminded by the weight of the broken dreams that seemed to impress on me the knowledge that my grief could not be alleviated by such superficial activity. My period of mourning continued off and on for many years, as the layers of loss after divorce are unexpectedly far-reaching, extending to painful reconfigurations between shared friends and in-laws and even to the grudging acceptance of a new spouse who would also share our child. What I also learned was that the values associated with the paradigms of marriage and family, so deeply ingrained in my consciousness, were difficult to alter. The loss of an identity that was socially acceptable made me feel painfully aware of being a misfit in my own community. With no foundation to anchor me, I felt that I was dangling, drifting like an alien in an unfamiliar world, just "I, and Silence, some strange Race / Wrecked, solitary, here" (J280/Fr340). "Wrecked" and "solitary" described perfectly the way I saw my condition.

In an effort to immerse myself in a familiar and much-loved activity that would distract me from my conflicted state of mind and provide some kind of secure footing, I enrolled in an American literature class, where I was introduced to Emily Dickinson's poetry. I felt an immediate and intimate connection with this nineteenth-century poet. I found her work to be so intellectually challenging, so psychologically insightful and emotionally intense, that my psyche was both provoked and nourished by her language. The compelling power of its "truth" awakened and focused me, pointed me with optimism towards a new path, and lifted me out of the dreary and unending landscape of melancholy in which I had been living. More importantly, at that emotionally difficult and confusing time, Dickinson's poetry became as alive and real as a wise companion—in truth, a spiritual guide—to whom I could guiltlessly turn whenever I needed but who thankfully did not require anything from me. In spite of Dickinson's acute awareness that we must pursue our healing process alone, as she states in a letter to Mrs. Holland, saying, "There are depths in every Consciousness, from which we cannot rescue ourselves — to which none can go with us — which represent to us Mortally — the Adventure of Death" (L555), she, by virtue of her presence in language, was and still is with me.

Even now, as I return to the lines that both terrified and attracted me at the outset of my painful journey, I feel the impact of Dickinson's powerful words and the difficult truth they hold.

> To fill a Gap
> Insert the Thing that caused it —
> Block it up
> With Other — and 'twill yawn the more —
> You cannot solder an Abyss
> With Air — (J546/Fr647)

Another partner, another marriage, I dreamed, would assuage the wound that divorce inflicted, but deep down I knew that what was lost was irrecoverable: the dream of a happy and lifelong relationship, the dream of a whole family, the dream of providing the best home environment for my young child, the dream of the supportive network of shared friends and extended family. The truth of Dickinson's words rang with great clarity in my mind, expressing distinctly what had been only inchoate emotion within me: "You cannot solder an Abyss / With Air"—the "Abyss," I thought, must be that uncomfortable rush of adrenaline that made my stomach clench; the "Air," the insufficient substitutions with which I tried to fill the gaps in my life. But, even though I knew that the wound was permanent, instead of being disturbed, I felt a strange kind of comfort in Dickinson's bold statement of another disarming truth:

> They say that "Time assuages" —
> Time never did assuage —
> An actual suffering strengthens
> As Sinews do, with Age —
>
> Time is a Test of Trouble —
> But not a Remedy —
> If such it prove, it prove too
> There was no Malady — (J686/Fr861)

If this poem asserted the truth of the matter, I asked myself, then where could I find hope that my pain would lessen, that I would return to life and trust the future again? Or, indeed, how could I see any value in the pain I was feeling? Hoping to find an answer to that question in her poems, I turned in earnest to my studies. However, finding that answer wasn't quite as easy as I might have expected. Dickinson's method of consolation, a byproduct of her own process of healing, lies somewhat covertly expressed in her characteristic practice of "slant truth-telling" whereby she guides and "teaches" us using nondidactic methods. For, despite her clear intent to console, stated most overtly in the sentimentality of "If I can stop one Heart from Breaking" (J919/Fr982), and, with more complexity, in another poem where she claims that the act of "saving" is an "Art" that should be the obligation of those who survive, she deliberately leaves the sufferer alone to carry out her own journey of self-healing. However, throughout the poem, Dickinson does tell us a great deal about her method and intentions.

The Province of the Saved
Should be the Art — To Save —
Through Skill obtained in Themselves —
The Science of the Grave

No Man can understand
But He that hath endured
The Dissolution — in Himself —
That Man — be qualified

To qualify Despair
To Those who failing new —
Mistake Defeat for Death — Each time —
Till acclimated — to — (J539/Fr659)

It is very easy, she attests, for the despondent to "Mistake Defeat for death" and, giving up hope, to fail anew in the attempt to transcend the pain in order to live again. By capitalizing the first letter in the words "Despair" and "Death" and juxtaposing them in the third stanza, Dickinson emphasizes their contingency and foregrounds the gravity of the despair that makes us feel that life is over. But those who have gone through pain and are "Saved," who thus have the necessary experience (what she calls "The Science of the Grave," the knowledge derived from these deathlike periods of pain) and the necessary requirements to "qualify Despair," have come to recognize "Defeat" as temporary, not final, not "Death." Dickinson's play of words—between "qualified," to have the capacity, and "qualify," to modify or moderate—provides a link between the second and third stanzas, yet the contiguity of the root word foregrounds the interdependency of the two forms of the word. By arranging her words in this way, Dickinson emphasizes the interrelationship of the work we must do within ourselves and the transformation of consciousness that necessitates a kind of psychic death to life as we once knew it, what she might call "a Funeral, in [the] Brain" (J280/Fr340), that will ultimately lead to enlightenment and recovery. The end result of this qualifying process will not remove the pain (in truth, it cannot be removed), but it will mitigate it by changing our perception so that we become acclimated to our new conditions. But even as the poem asserts its point, the poet does not offer a procedure to be followed in the process of healing. We are only left to wonder how the poet who writes, "They say that 'Time assuages' — / Time never did assuage," who warns us against a passive faith in the belief of God's promise of an afterlife ("Narcotics cannot still the Tooth / That nibbles at the soul" [J501/Fr373]), and whose skepticism and equivocation offer no assurances has the capacity to provide us with much-needed consolation.

There is no question—and there is a great deal of scholarship to prove it—Dickinson's oeuvre constitutes an ongoing soul-searching project; Dickinson's brilliant insights into the condition of pain are evidence of her own losses, loneliness, and emotional conflicts. Her pain, however, enters the text obliquely, for the biographical elements do not constitute the *subject* of the poetry so much as its hermeneutics. The poet's language inscribes her awareness of the inescapable condition of human experience and is closely allied with the presence of the void, the underlying gap that informs the poet's elliptical expression. Sharon Cameron, in *Lyric Time*, emphasizes this association with the following observation: "Pain in Dickinson's poems is not always a feeling; it is sometimes presented in a spatial configuration, a blacking and blanking out. . . . Pain is the line drawn around a speaker's experience, separating her from vision, thought, and, above all, from the framing utterance. . . . Pain is the space where words would be, the hole torn out of language."[1] Moreover, in the many poems about suffering in the Dickinson canon, readers, struck by the lack of specific reference to the loss that might have inspired it, must, for the most part, allow that information to remain indeterminate, irrecoverable. As a result of such ellipsis, the reader's attention turns, in the end, away from the single biographical event to more universal considerations; that is, it turns to the effects of pain on human consciousness. And who has written more acutely on pain than Emily Dickinson? Many of the lines from her poignant poems are engraved in my mind: "There is a pain — so utter"

(J599/Fr515); "Pain — has an Element of Blank" (J650/Fr760); "After great pain, a formal feeling comes" (J341/Fr372); "Pain — expands the Time" (J967/Fr833). These and many more poems offered me the "liquid Word to make [my] sorrow less" (L859) simply because of the truth they expressed. I began to be aware of a certain pattern in Dickinson's writing: the compelling first lines that would pull me into the poem, trusting that I would find some kind of answer, some kind of anodyne to alleviate my pain, but then the poem would become more and more esoteric, often moving toward incomprehensibility. With time, I have come to see this as a deliberate method in that we follow the poet from the point of our present reality—feelings of acute pain—to an inward spiritual search of ourselves. Hardly aware at the time of what was happening, thinking that I was simply trying "to figure the poem out," I was actually doing something of far more personal significance; that is, I was executing a rigorous self-examination of all the dark corridors that the wound of divorce had forced me to enter. I began to understand that while the divorce itself was a distinct and painful rupture in my life, Dickinson's view of that rupture as a wound around which deeply significant meanings accrue began to lead me slowly toward accepting it. Quite simply, I began to feel a renewed hope.

The poet's philosophy that destabilization and disorientation brought on by pain create a new landscape in which there are no hierarchies, indeed, no frame of reference for authority or priority, thus presents an opportunity for new growth. We become acclimated, experiencing, as it were, a climate change in consciousness because of the very nature of imagination. As the poet Wallace Stevens writes, "[The imagination] is always attaching itself to a new reality, and adhering to it. It is not that there is a new imagination but that there is a new reality."[2] Thus, like Adrienne Rich's Madame Curie, whose "wounds came from the same place as her power,"[3] Dickinson's wounds and power become paradoxically interrelated. Her internalization of the underlying tensions between joy and pain, Eros and Thanatos, inscribed in oxymorons such as "Heavenly Hurt," "sumptuous Despair," and "sweet Torment," may account for the oracular and, indeed, consolatory power of her poetry. Dickinson's execution of oppositional stances emphasizes the space between as the site where we attempt to reach for our desires—where the acceptance of indeterminacy is crucial to our acceptance of the meaning of life itself. Just as the third chapter of Ecclesiastes asserts that contradictions are necessarily the basis of life, so Dickinson emphasizes the paradoxical truth and the richness of experience that emerges from opposing states. But it takes considerable time—at least it did for me—to embrace an entirely new way of looking at the function of pain in our lives. It's a slowly evolving process that leads toward understanding Dickinson's idea that "Power is only Pain — / Stranded, thro' Discipline" (J252/Fr312).

In Michael Richardson's critical biography of Georges Bataille, he notes Bataille's insights into his own inner journey as a wisdom that is shamanistic in its spirituality and that can only be gained by exploring the limits of experience, through pain or sickness even to death itself: "The essence of the experience of shamanism lies in the wound, in the terrible wound that opens up being. One could only become a shaman through being sick and following the path of sickness to its limit, to its substantiality, which is death. To become a shaman one had to cure oneself by a confrontation with death." [4] The rigors of soul-making demand that we face the pain, go through it, not around it: we must take, as Dickinson says, "the old road through pain." Thus, in those experiences that wound us, we experience what the poet describes in "There's a certain slant of light"—an oxymoronic "Heavenly Hurt" for which "We can find no scar / But internal difference / Where the Meanings, are" (J258/F320). In Dickinson's text, gaps and ellipses are the fissures, the sites of wounds, the multiply constructed oppositions that go far beyond conventional literary devices yet arise from them. Opposites become undifferentiated, their "difference" glimpsed only through the seams. In the end, what is described as the destruction of an order is really the destruction of *seeing* that order. Dickinson's consolatory purpose would appear to be in active play since she must defend herself against external forces that would sabotage her project.

Ultimately, she succeeds in turning her pain into power, a point that Joanne Feit Diehl aptly summarizes in her canonical essay "'Ransom in a Voice': Language as Defense in Dickinson's Poetry."

> Dickinson imbues her poetic enterprise with a vision of language operating as defense against the pressures of rejection and exile that define her world. Here is a definition of poetry that possesses, like Blake's visionary language, the capacity to mold the terms of existence within the fires of her own imagination. Such a vision of language originates in the perceived absence of external allies and the poet's compensatory devotion not to the conditions of the world, but, instead, to what Dickinson called the "Art within the Soul" (J855/Fr1091).[5]

Such is our own mission, as well—to own the art within our souls—to "mold the terms of existence within the fires of" our own imaginations in the intensely complex process of soul-making. Fittingly, according to psychologist

James Hillman in *Healing Fiction,* the work of the soul operates necessarily on poetic terms.

> The essence of word-images is that they are free from the perceptible world and free one from it. They take the mind home, to its poetic base, to the imaginal. . . . If we are ill because of these intolerable images, we get well because of imagination. Poesis as therapy. . . . They present us with the chance to recognize ourselves in the mess of the world as having been engaged and always being engaged in soul-making, where "making" returns to its original meaning of *poesis,* the making of soul through the imagination of words.[6]

The shifting notion of the self necessarily precludes stasis; the "center" itself is subject to both collapse and renewal, an idea that Dickinson describes in this poem about soul-making.

Each Life Converges to some Centre —
Expressed — or still —
Exists in every Human Nature
A Goal —

Embodied scarcely to itself — it may be —
Too fair
For Credibility's presumption
To mar —

Adored with caution — as a Brittle Heaven —
To reach
Were hopeless, as the Rainbow's Raiment
To touch —

Yet persevered toward — surer — for the Distance —
How high —
Unto the Saints' slow diligence —
The Sky —

Ungained — it may be — by a Life's low Venture —
But then —
Eternity enable the endeavoring
Again. (J680/Fr724)

The poet destabilizes, indeed de-centers, the meaning of the word "Centre," so that it becomes as dynamic as the process of working toward it. The process of persevering toward a goal is shown to resist linearity by raising the possibility that it may not even be expressed, though latent, "still." Even the expression of a goal leaves it in an extremely fragile position, as the crabbed syntax suggests. Therefore, the only certainty we have of knowing it is provided by its distance from us, "yet — Persevered toward — surer — for the Distance." The poem— like life itself—moves in both directions, outward and inward, from and to a center that is neither fixed nor defined but as certain as our own existence. We must change as the conditions of our lives change.

Thus Dickinson's ongoing quest is limitless, extending even after life, an idea she raises in letter 650, in which she speaks of her conversations with Austin about "the Extension of Consciousness." As Hillman asserts, "Know Thyself is its own end and has no end. It is Mercurial. It is a paradoxical hermetic art that is both goal-directed and without end. . . . There is no other end than the act of soul-making itself and soul is without end."[7] In a parallel way, the cut or seam of the wounded text, in turn, creates a longing in the reader, a longing for the presence of the poet herself—or at least a presence that is representative of de-terminacy—which also causes pain because we can never succeed in attaining it. Therefore, as Robert McClure Smith points out in *The Seductions of Emily Dickinson,* our attention turns to the glistening, "fleshly" surface of the words themselves, the trace of what is irrecoverably lost.

> Although as readers we cannot immediately recover the lost presence, we can still sense its lingering trace, there, at a remove, distanced by space and time. Presence tantalizes through the seductive suggestion of its possible recovery. Of course, ultimately, presence cannot be detected by its trace, because that trace is merely another absence, another sign that can designate presence only by virtue of its differing *from* that presence. As such, presence can never be recovered. But the *illusion* that it actually can be recovered is the perpetual motor of our reading desire, a desire for the complete possession that could heal the more fundamental difference within.[8]

And the trace lies, can only lie, in the language itself. Wallace Stevens sees the potent power of the poet as having the ability to provide the necessary resources to bring us through dark times, saying that "the deepening need for words to express our thoughts and feelings which, we are sure, are all the truth that we shall ever experience, having no illusions, makes us listen to words when we hear them, loving them and feeling them, makes us search the sound of them, for a finality, a perfection, an unalterable vibration, which it is only within the power of the acutest poet to give them."[9] Stevens's focus on the consolatory power of the word itself emphasizes the materiality of language, or what Brenda Ludeman describes as the Kristevan notion of the "textual and palpable status of language—a physical presence given as other to signification" to which we respond.[10] Trusting in the "truth" conveyed by the "corporeality" of the text is crucial both to the psychological recovery of the reader and to the survival of the poet. The reader's existential need for the utterance of feeling, feeling then discovered in the "body" of the text that also in*corp*orates the writer's body, makes us work to fill the gap that exists between one solitary soul and another—between now and eternity—to find the trace in the words to which we can bond, to attach ourselves so that we, too, may participate in the infinite and be consoled by the greater truths of those spheres.

Dickinson's own professed "life in language" informs her rhetorical strategies as she inscribes all these ideas into a kind of semiotic synaesthesia. The talismanic effect of her words, carrying a heavy freight of meaning that continues to expand throughout her work, is reassuring. We can hold onto something—hold it like a rosary bead, repeat it like a mantra, each time returning to it in our minds, on our tongues, in a way that increases its value and brings it into ourselves. In this way, like the privileging of signifiers that are connected and yet simultaneously held apart and kept together by the dashes, "the body [—her body—] can be 'lifted' into a language that aspires to the mimesis of materiality."[11]

So when Dickinson writes to Mrs. Henry Hills that "the power to console is not within corporeal reach—though its' attempt, is precious" (L596), we come to see that the poet's "attempt" lies in the very numinosity of her language that draws us to her and heightens our longing to possess her, to seek comfort in her Truth. We do not touch her, but we are touched, soulfully, by her language. But the unknown, according to Dickinson, "is the largest need of the intellect" (L559) and so we must lose her body and the determinacy it represents in order to gain ourselves. The work of healing is a solitary process, but the consolation that Dickinson brings to us lies in her very attempt to help and, most of all, in the rich potency of her words, which encourage our ability to see "possibilities" once again.

· · ·

For over twenty years now, my connection to Emily Dickinson has been as personal as it has been scholarly. And in many ways, I think that Dickinson's project has been similarly composed. Her life is inscribed in her words, yet despite the intimate glimpse we have into her soul, we will never know the specifics of that singular life. She wants it that way. Like any great mentor or shaman, she deflects the glory from herself, knowing that her words, her Art, will hold a power sufficient to endure, to influence, and, certainly, to heal.

The wound we experience opens us up to a place where boundaries are dissolved, where the oppositions we normally see as separate become intermingled. In fact, we enter a spiritual dimension that, as disorienting and painful as it might be, has the capacity to bring us enlightenment and peace. But, a word of caution: it is within our power to make sense of the pain, to be liberated from it; however, if we cannot, we continue to be imprisoned by it. It's all in the mind: "Captivity is Consciousness — So's Liberty" (J384/Fr649). Thus the wound becomes the site of profound significance, with the power to integrate and connect us rather than to fragment and isolate us, but the journey requires the utmost patience and solitude.

> Growth of Man — like Growth of Nature —
> Gravitates within —
> Atmosphere, and Sun endorse it —
> But it stir — alone —
>
> Each — it's difficult Ideal
> Must achieve — Itself —
> Through the solitary prowess
> Of a Silent Life —
>
> Effort — is the sole condition —
> Patience of Itself —
> Patience of opposing forces —
> And intact Belief —
>
> Looking on — is the Department
> Of it's Audience —
> But Transaction — is assisted
> By no Countenance — (J750/Fr790)

As time passes, retrospect teaches us to see the moment of crisis with wiser, more accepting and compassionate eyes so that "'Tis good—the looking back on Grief" because even "though the Woe you have Today / Be larger — As the Sea," it "Exceeds it's Unremembered Drop — / They're Water — equally" (J660/Fr472).

The truth, of course, is that the wound never heals—not completely—but we can become acclimated to living with it, to seeing it as one drop in the oceanic sphere of our psyche, of our spirit. But with Dickinson's guidance, I have come to see that it is even possible to "love the wound" because it has been the site of such significance in my life—to my soul—that I have even come to be grateful for it, with the humility that Dickinson expresses when she writes, "Joy to have merited the Pain" (J788/Fr739). And that lesson, perhaps, is what brought the wilderness of the unfamiliar world into which pain had thrown me—flung me, as Dickinson might say—at last to a state of Peace—to where I "own the Art within [my] Soul" (J855/Fr1091) and have swept and scoured the darker corridors of the psyche to emerge stronger, more self-reliant, and more in tune with myself—indeed, to at last know myself. When we think of Dickinson's exhortation, "Soto! Explore thyself!" (J832/Fr814), we know that she has been on that very mission. To be true to one's self, to live life authentically—*that* is the Art we are all capable of creating—to make an Art of our lives. That was the pearl for which Dickinson was so fervently diving, fathoms deep where the "Sea / Develop[s] Pearl, and Weed" (J732/Fr857). That was the pearl for which I, too, was searching—submerged as it was under the weeds of self-deception and inauthenticity. I know now that my divorce wasn't the sole cause of my pain. It was symptomatic of a much deeper malaise that was aching for me to rigorously explore myself, to heal myself, so that I would find a power based on self-knowledge and self-love and to finally be able to claim as triumphantly as Dickinson, "On a Columnar Self — How ample — to rely " (J789/Fr740).

> It ceased to hurt me, though so slow
> I could not feel the Anguish go —
> But only knew by looking back —
> That something — had benumbed the Track —
>
> Nor when it altered, I could say,
> For I had worn it, every day,
> As constant as the Childish frock —
> I hung upon the Peg, at night.
>
> But not the Grief — that nestled close
> As needles — ladies softly press
> To Cushions Cheeks —
> To keep their place —

Nor what consoled it, I could trace —
Except, whereas 'twas Wilderness
It's better — almost Peace — (J584/Fr421)

Notes

1. Sharon Cameron, *Lyric Time: Dickinson and the Limits of Genre* (Baltimore and London: Johns Hopkins Univ. Press, 1992), 158.

2. Wallace Stevens, "The Noble Rider and the Sound of Words," in *The Necessary Angel: Essays on Reality and the Imagination* (New York: Vintage Books, 1965), 22.

3. Adrienne Rich, "Power," in *Dream of a Common Language: Poems 1974–1977* (New York: W. W. Norton, 1978).

4. Michael Richardson, *Georges Bataille* (London: Routledge, 1994), 114.

5. Joanne Feit Diehl, "'Ransom in a Voice': Language as Defense in Dickinson's Poetry," in *Feminist Critics Read Emily Dickinson*, ed. Suzanne Juhasz (Bloomington: Indiana Univ. Press, 1983).

6. James Hillman, *Healing Fiction* (Woodstock: Spring Publications, 1983), 47–49.

7. Ibid., 80–81.

8. Robert McClure Smith, *The Seductions of Emily Dickinson* (Tuscaloosa: Univ. of Oklahoma Press, 1996), 128.

9. Stevens, 32.

10. Brenda Ludeman, "Julia Kristeva: The Other Side of Language," in *The Judgement of Paris: Recent French Theory in a Local Context,* ed. Kevin D. S. Murray (North Sydney: Allen and Unwin, 1992), 23–37.

11. Smith, 128.

Broken Silence

The Healing Power of Emily Dickinson's Poetry

SUSAN HESS

For more than forty years, the clandestine events of my childhood and young adulthood were known only to me and to my abusers. But in April 2005, I displayed an exhibit of woven tapestries that interpret twenty-four of Emily Dickinson's poems. Her words and my tapestries openly tell the story of my abuse as well as my personal journey of healing. For me, the exhibition was the psychological equivalent of delivering the eulogy at my own funeral as I celebrated my emergence from behind a wall of secrecy.

After randomly selecting a poem from her collection at our town library, the first Emily Dickinson poem I read articulated exactly what I had experienced: years of childhood abuse.

> That sacred Closet when you sweep —
> Entitled "Memory" —
> Select a reverential Broom —
> And do it silently.
>
> 'Twill be a Labor of surprise —
> Besides Identity
> Of other Interlocutors
> A probability —
>
> August the Dust of that Domain —
> Unchallenged — let it lie —
> You cannot supersede itself
> But it can silence you — (J1273/Fr1385)

All citations of Dickinson's poems used in this chapter are from *The Poems of Emily Dickinson,* ed. Thomas H. Johnson, 3 vols. (Cambridge, Mass.: Harvard Univ. Press, 1955).

60

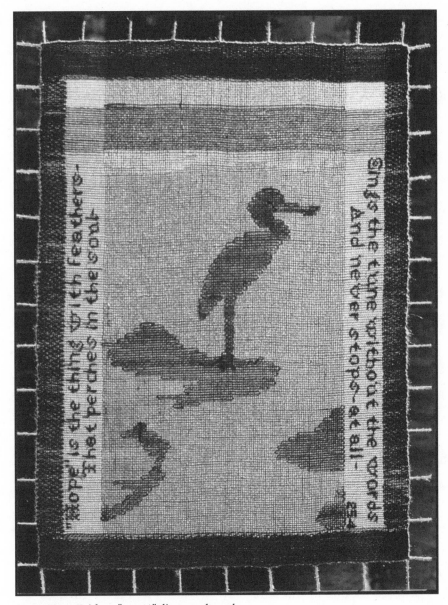

Susan Hess, *Faith.* 20" x 15¼", linen and wool.

Throughout many years of therapy, I had been silently and reverentially sweeping my memory. Reading her work, the dust of my past could no longer silence me as my voice began to express with confidence an identity along the journey upon which I was about to embark.

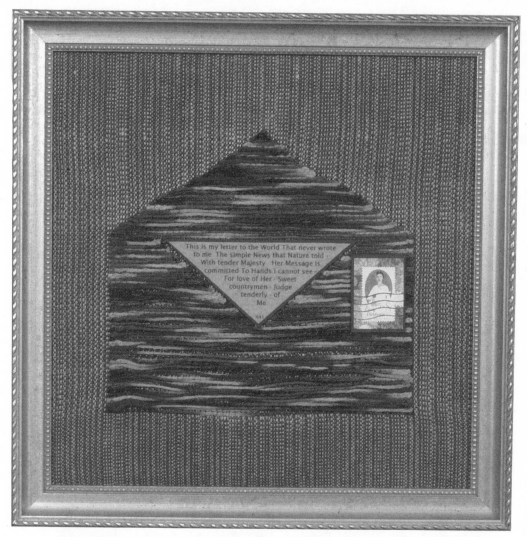

Susan Hess, *Prologue.* 15" x 15", linen and silk.

As I read Dickinson, I intuitively became aware that a new method of self-exploration was revealed to me. She perceived and explored states of psychological processes and explained experiences and emotions that mirrored my own. As though she were speaking through me, I could identify the same emotions. I was especially intrigued by the poet's architectural images. She assigned fragments of memory to specific areas in the house—the front, the rear, the attic, the windows, the doors. These images provided access to my own spontaneous, creative imagination; reconnection to the uninhibited expressions of my childhood; and, most importantly, a path to freedom. As though she were speaking to me, I could identify the shame of my past, my unresolved grief, my renegade spiritual beliefs, my fears, my silence, and my wounded soul.

Dickinson believed that truth could heal the human spirit. Her lyrics leapt from the page to meet my mental and emotional needs and transformed me. Her weaving of words and my weaving of threads represent the way in which art has the capacity to heal. The twenty-four tapestries I've woven to illustrate Dickinson's poems follow my own journey of healing from *Discovery,* to *Acceptance,* and finally to *Freedom.*

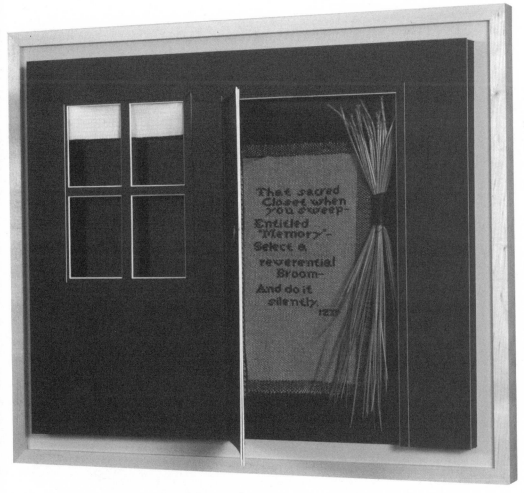

Susan Hess, *Healing.* 19" x 23", linen and cotton.

I believe Emily Dickinson was a master craftswoman whose poetry was an art of transformation, just as my weavings are for me. I was a victim, but because of Dickinson's genius, I am a survivor and have found the courage and resolve to carry my message to abuse victims and survivors who continue to suffer.

NOTE

Illustrations of all of Susan's work can be found in her self-published collection *"I'm Nobody": A Journal of Healing. Weaving Truth with Trust* (2004).

Hope and the Flight of
United Airlines 232, July 1989

Mell McDonnell

Footage of the plane cartwheeling over in flames and smoke plays over and over in my mind when I close my eyes. We've seen it now so many times. First at the Air National Guard Armory only one hour after the crash, then at the hospital, and continually in the common room of the college where we're staying now.

How could I have survived it?

United 232 from Denver is an easy, just-another-business-trip flight. Sitting comfortably on the plane, I'm writing a script and thinking I rather like the beginning. Then, an hour after departure, there is a soft, thud-like explosion. The big DC-10 shudders, and all 298 of us simultaneously draw in our collective breath and say, "My God! What was that!?"

The captain instantly comes on the intercom, "Folks, that was one engine that just blew. We're going to be a little late getting into Chicago."

I feel fear high in my throat, but Shauna Brown, the chief stewardess, remains calm, and my seatmate is talking about how they can bring these planes down on one engine. When we start to drift downward, he says that we're going lower to go slower. I believe him—although I don't, really.

Old prayers, old poems, and thoughts of my family—my family—my family race through my head. What's the right way to die? Don't Cheyenne have words to chant in order to pass through the doors of death? I know these are not idle questions. An Emily Dickinson poem rises to the surface.

"Hope" is the thing with feathers —
That perches in the soul —
And sings the song without the words —
And never stops — at all. . . .

All citations of Dickinson's poems used in this chapter are from *The Poems of Emily Dickinson,* ed. Thomas H. Johnson, 3 vols. (Cambridge, Mass.: Harvard Univ. Press, 1955).

The rhythms buoy me up. The soft sounds and the long and short vowels gently touching one another fill my heart, my entire body, and ease my terror. I hold onto the long *o* in "Hope" as if it were a life preserver.

> And sweetest — in the Gale — is heard
> And sore must be the storm —
> That could abash the little Bird
> That kept so many warm. . . .

The worst is yet to come—is happening now—and I cling to the words. They are my only shield against annihilation. If I say them, I cannot not be.

For twenty-five minutes, the plane slews from side to side, losing altitude, banking first this way, then that. Every time it turns, it drones lazily like a biplane on a summer afternoon. I think of John Wayne whistling "The High and the Mighty." But the words are my ballast. Are they a talisman against the void—or an entry into it? I can't ponder that now, and strangely it does not seem to matter.

Now the captain again: "We're landing in Sioux City, Iowa, in about ten minutes. I won't hide it from you. It's going to be rough. I'll tell you to brace three times, just before touching down." We read the seat-pocket card and listen to the stewardess as we've never listened before.

Five more sickening minutes.

"Brace! Brace! Brace!" the captain screams. We throw ourselves down, arms crossed, clutching ankles, eyes squeezed shut. I press my face into my bare knees and breathe deep.

There's a terrible lashing about—a chaos of doors and windows moving and heaving—King Kong shaking the tower. Space is totally transformed.

Blackness.

I'm hanging upside down. The floor is the ceiling. I suck in my breath, and in one gymnastic gesture flip the buckle on my seat belt and land on my feet.

Two steps. I'm stopped by wires. There's heat and smoke on the left side. I cannot die now. *"Hope" is the thing with feathers.* . . . I carefully lift each foot and file after other passengers into a green light. How can the cargo hold be so full of foliage? I'm mistaken. It's corn. We're in a cornfield!

I'm running straight down a row—faster, faster. *And never stops—at all.* . . . People from the back pass me. I slip into another row and keep a steady pace. The corn blades are sharp, hard, emerald green scythes. It's like running a gauntlet. Is this what combat's like? *And sweetest — in the Gale — is heard.* . . .

Here's a country road up on something like a berm or a levee. I come up from the ocean's bottom, scarcely winded, just blowing out hard. Behind me, a sea of green with heads bobbing in it. *I've heard it in the chillest land — / And on the strangest Sea. . . .* Everyone on the road is shouting, "Come away, come away from the plane. It's going to blow up!"

Here's a stewardess herding passengers like baby chicks. I hold and pat a young blonde girl who's sobbing hysterically. She's trembling and crying, and then her whole family—all seven of them—come out of the rows and I give her to them. Other families are coming together now.

A pretty Asian girl, her face deepening to what looks like a bad sunburn, stands there, her singed hair clinging to her face. I turn her into the wind and carefully pick each strand from her skin.

Back there, black, acrid smoke spirals up. We can't see much. Streams of water like squirts from a toy water pistol play against it.

Around us, it's a summer day in Iowa. The faint, not unpleasant odor of dairy cows floats over the corn, birds are singing, the sun is warm on our hands and faces. All of us are thirsty.

Five minutes pass, then ten, then fifteen. Finally, a blue school bus comes jolting up the road. We're loaded on. It grinds gears, lurches forward, and within minutes, we see it—the fuselage, the engine, the tail section scattered like a huge broken carcass. My seatmate says that she sees bodies all bluish and twisted among the strewn wreckage. I don't look.

Then a volunteer says that I should go to the hospital. The paramedic who takes us calls us "the walking wounded," which strikes me as strangely funny. The rest of the afternoon is a blur of doctors' exams—I have full range of motion in all joints—phone calls—finally I reach my mother—and so many solicitous hands and voices.

It'll be this way for the next twenty-four hours. We're touched and consoled and asked to talk, and told that we don't have to talk, and asked how we've slept or if we've slept. So many kind, simple gestures and sympathetic faces. So many professional people hoping to say the right thing at the right time.

I want to be alone, to walk barefoot in the grass, to look at the light. It can't be done. The media are everywhere. Even they, beyond their hunger for a story, look young and human and alive. And that, we all hold in common.

> I've heard it in the chillest land —
> And on the strangest Sea —
> Yet, never, in Extremity,
> It asked a crumb — of Me.

. . .

The crash of United Airlines 232 in Sioux City, Iowa, was said to be the second-worst crash in U.S. aviation history. The plane was a DC-10 with a capacity of 350. When it crashed on Wednesday, July 19, 1989, around 4 P.M., it was carrying an estimated 287 passengers and 11 crew members. Newspaper accounts from the next day reported that 125, including one of the stewardesses, died. The captain's name was Al Haynes. He was just about to retire, and his experience was credited with saving as many lives as he did.

I was sitting in row 10-C, a couple of rows behind the bulkhead and close to the aisle on the inside, which was fortunate for me because the fire broke out on the outside of the plane. I was spared being scorched. Rows 9 through 23 in the plane were comparatively intact. Most who died were seated below row 23 or forward in first class. The fire and police departments of Sioux City had just completed disaster training and drill the previous week and were completely prepared to put out the fire, treat the wounded, and house the rest of us. I got back on a plane the following day around 3 P.M. and flew back to Denver. I remain unafraid to fly.

May the Circle Be Unbroken

Reading Emily Dickinson after 9/11

ELLEN LOUISE HART

The Poets light but
Lamps —
Themselves — go out —
The Wicks they
stimulate —
If vital Light

Inhere as do the
Suns —
Each Age a Lens
Disseminating their
Circumference — [1]

The mission statement of the Emily Dickinson Museum, in Amherst, Massachusetts, asserts its dedication "to educate diverse audiences about Emily Dickinson's life, family, creative work, times, and enduring relevance."[2] The role that Dickinson's poems have played on a national stage during the tragic events at the start of the twenty-first century are testimony to that "enduring relevance." As Americans grieved the September 11, 2001, attacks and the subsequent U.S. invasion of Iraq, as the war in Iraq continues and the political divide over the future of our democracy widens, Dickinson's poems have been at the center of public events bringing people together to mourn our losses, to give voice to our fears, and to reach out to find comfort and courage.

In the context of these historical events, four Dickinson poems in particular were chosen by readers to console, illuminate, and inspire. The first is "After great pain, a formal feeling comes," mailed out by the Dickinson Homestead advisory committee in their first newsletter after September 11; the second,

"Much Madness is divinest Sense," had to be on our minds after a White House symposium on American poetry was cancelled, as the United States prepared to invade Iraq, and as Poets Against the War held protest readings around the country; the third, "Revolution is the Pod," helped me respond to militarism and threats to our democracy; and the last poem, "A little Madness in the Spring," provided the title for a week of events in the spring of 2004 at the Emily Dickinson Museum that included a marathon-style community reading of Dickinson's poetry. During such times of darkness and transition, as readers circle around each other in grief and in recovery, Dickinson's poems serve as lamps "disseminating their Circumference."

AFTER GREAT PAIN, A FORMAL FEELING COMES —

After the attacks on September 11, readers began posting and circulating poems of mourning. "Almost immediately after the event, improvised memorials, often conceived around poems, sprang up all over the city," writes *New York Times* correspondent Dinitia Smith.[3] She describes the tragic scene at Ground Zero, the "bits of famous poems, original poems, snatches of verse pinned alongside photos of the victims." During those first days and weeks, readers e-mailed poems to friends, family, and colleagues. The most widely distributed was W. H. Auden's "September 1, 1939."

Auden writes of a man in a bar in New York contemplating the invasion of Poland by Germany; the man is deeply dissatisfied with the way he has conducted his life and overwhelmed by confusion and guilt. In September 2001, we found extraordinary parallels in Auden's lines.

> Waves of anger and fear
> Circulate over the bright
> And darkened lands of the earth,
> Obsessing our private lives;
> The unmentionable odour of death
> Offends the September night. . . . [4]

In "The News from Poetry," journalist Margo Jefferson writes that "poetry can be the only sure conduit to emotional truths that politics has done its best to shut down."[5] And the penultimate stanza of Auden's poem reflects that thought: "All I have is a voice / To undo the folded lie. . . . We must love one another or die."

After September 11, readers were looking for images of people surviving the shock and grief, then making a commitment to live by their conscience. The front matter of Neil Astley's 2002 anthology, *Staying Alive: Real Poems for Unreal Times,* pairs Dickinson's criterion for recognizing poetry ("If I read a book [and] it makes my whole body so cold no fire ever can warm me I know *that* is poetry") with Kafka's criterion for prose ("A book must be the axe which smashes the frozen sea within us.")[6] Living in the presence of the forces of creativity is essential, as we try, in Astley's words, "to make sense of a new age of information and double-speak, technology and terrorism, of war and world poverty."[7]

In the Dickinson Homestead advisory committee's quarterly publication of fall 2001, the editors offered a "reflection" poem.[8]

After great pain, a formal
feeling comes —
The Nerves sit ceremonious,
 like Tombs —
The stiff Heart questions 'Was
 it He, that bore,'
And 'Yesterday, or 'Centuries before'?

The Feet, mechanical, go round —
Of Ground, or Air, or Ought —
A Wooden way
Regardless grown,
A Quartz contentment, like
 a stone —

This is the Hour of Lead —
Remembered, if outlived,
As Freezing persons, recollect
 the Snow —
First — chill — then stupor — then
 the letting go —

A message followed this poem: "As this newsletter goes to press, we are just comprehending the magnitude of the events that occurred in the United States on Tuesday, September 11. During this time, we hope that Dickinson's poems speak to you in your efforts to cope, to remember, to recover."

Cartoonist Lynda Barry chose the same poem that September for her strip, "Ernie Pook's Comeek." In the first of four frames, a teenage girl, Maybonne Mullens, sits in her house at the bottom of a staircase. She is dressed in a nightgown with stars on it and looks sad and pensive; the first stanza of Dickinson's poem is printed above the scene. In the next box, a close-up of the same scene, Maybonne looks sad and frightened; the poem's second stanza appears above. In frame 3, under the last stanza of the poem, Maybonne looks sad and tired, as if she were somewhere far away, not noticing that her younger sister Marlys is approaching. In the final frame, Marlys, wearing a striped nightgown, wraps her arms around Maybonne, comforting her wiser, tougher sister. Stars and stripes, the nightgown patterns, are united. Marlys's stripes are angled toward the top of the stairs behind her, which suggests that things are looking up. Cir-

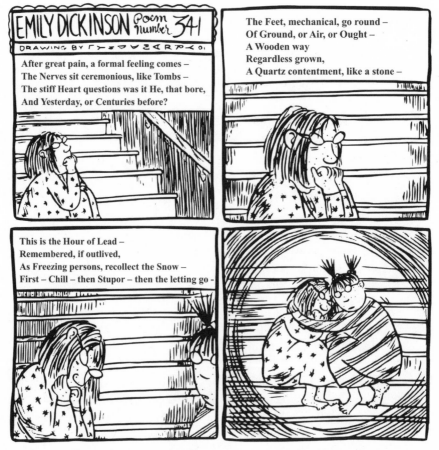

Lynda Barry, from Salon.com, September 21, 2001. Reprinted with permission.

cles within circles are drawn around the sisters, like lenses letting Marlys and Maybonne look out and readers look in. The message is that all of us can reach out, hold on, and let go.

Some people read "After great pain, a formal / feeling comes" as a story of letting go of life, or letting go of sanity and descending into unconsciousness, madness, or despair. But Dickinson reader Lois Kaufman, serving as a volunteer grief counselor in the late 1990s with Front Porch, an organization in Atlanta for families who have lost a child, told me in an e-mail message that she found this poem useful in her work: "My second Front Porch session was Tuesday when I was asked to take the parents. It was a very productive session and when I shared 'After great pain,' they were completely at home with it. It was viewed, I believe, as rather a nuts-and-bolts expression of reality."

The poem makes a number of points that are characteristic of Dickinson's "thought," a term that she and other nineteenth-century writers, including Emerson and Thomas Wentworth Higginson, use to describe their writing. One of these characteristics is the exploration of a divided consciousness in which one part of the self, detached, watches and studies another part of the self. A second, as implausible as it may seem here, is that Dickinson looks at pain with humor. Third, the poet has faith that life, like nature, is a constant source of change. Regardless of a despair that threatens to obliterate consciousness, natural transitions—time, seasons, light, weather—continue. These changes provide impetus for incremental shifts in thought and feeling.

To trace nuances of meaning, I want to see the visual aspects of a Dickinson poem, the shapes and arrangements of lines and stanzas, the details of what I view as an expressive script. Therefore, I read in manuscript, which means that in place of standard print editions, whenever possible, I use images of the manuscript pages—photo reproductions or electronic images. Much of Dickinson's work exists in manuscript, though only transcripts or printed texts remain for some poems. I find that features of the handwritten text—line divisions; spacing around words and phrases; size and appearance of certain letters; length, angle, and position of dashes and other marks of punctuation—create visual effects that represent sound, interact with meter and rhythm, suggest emphasis, and create meaning. All Dickinson poems in this essay appear in print translations I have made from images of the poems in manuscript. Elsewhere I argue extensively for this kind of reading; here I model it, hoping to show its richness and productivity.

For example, the divided metrical line, "After great pain, a formal / feeling comes," slows the pace of the poem's opening and highlights the lofty expression. The line division draws attention to connections in meaning made through sound structure, particularly through alliteration: the pause created by the line break places extra stress on "feeling," enhancing the consonance of "formal," "feeling," "after," and "stiff." Nerves that once ruled "formally," "ceremoniously," make way for a "stiff Heart" to pose questions. As the poem goes on, forms become flexible. The language of the beginning gives way to more natural-sounding speech. Time starts up again: although the heart can't recognize when the trauma began or how long it lasted, in the poem's last stanza an hour is measured. Meter is varied. Dickinson puns on "feet," metrical feet and the two feet standing for the body as a whole: "The Feet, mechanical, go round — / Of Ground, or Air, or Ought." The second line can be read mechanically, monotonously, as if body and mind moved by rote.

In the final stanza, feelings soften and warm by degrees. Lead is softer than quartz. When skies are leaden and snow is about to fall, the temperature of air rises. The last two visual lines emphasize the culminating phrase by placing it on a line by itself: "the letting go." True rhyme for the last two metrical lines of each of the three stanzas creates a series that strengthens the poem's closure. Parts remembered and recollected make a whole person. "Freezing persons" is plural. She recognizes that she is not alone, that other people, too, have survived, coped, recovered. Then and now, knowing that other readers on the Dickinson Homestead mailing list and other fans of "Ernie Pook's Comeek" were experiencing the poem in a similar way and at the same time reminds me of circles to which we all belong.

Much Madness is divinest Sense

On February 12, 2003, Abraham Lincoln's birthday, First Lady Laura Bush, a former teacher and school librarian, scheduled a symposium on "Poetry and the American Voice" to be held at the White House. Discussion would focus on Dickinson, Walt Whitman, and Langston Hughes. Among the poets and literary scholars Mrs. Bush invited to participate was Sam Hamill, poet, editor, cofounder of Copper Canyon Press, and a former Marine who became a conscientious objector. The United States was preparing to invade Iraq, and the day after receiving his invitation, Hamill wrote fifty poet-friends that the "only legitimate response to such a morally bankrupt and unconscionable idea" as the proposed "Shock and Awe" attack on Baghdad was "to reconstitute a Poets Against the War movement," similar to artists' protests of the war in Vietnam.[9] Each poet was asked to send a poem to a Web site where the submissions would be organized, then printed out and presented to Laura Bush at the symposium. Hamill also asked his friends to circulate the message to others. Within four days, he received fifteen hundred poems. Hearing of Hamill's plan, the White House immediately "postponed" the gathering. A spokesperson for Laura Bush declared that "it would be inappropriate to turn a literary event into a political forum."[10]

Hamill's subsequent anthology, *Poets Against the War,* includes 262 of the poems collected, along with several "Statements of Conscience" that the writers were also invited to submit. Dickinson's work figured prominently in these statements. Robert Pinsky, former U.S. poet laureate and director of the Favorite Poem Project, in declining his invitation to attend the symposium, sent the White House the following message: "To participate in a poetry symposium that speaks of 'the' American voice, in the house of authority I mistrust, on the verge of a questionable war, is impossible—the more so when I remember the candid, rebellious, individualistic voices of Dickinson, Whitman, and Hughes."[11] Later Hamill echoed Pinsky in a message posted on the Poets Against the War Web site: "It remains for us to imagine a government grounded in compassionate policies toward its citizenry and toward the community of nations, a country that clings to democratic principles and counts every vote. It is for us to claim a great tradition of American poetry, to reinvigorate those democratic vistas and self-revelations Whitman and Dickinson bequeathed us, the social conscience Langston Hughes embodied."[12]

In the winter of 2003 Hamill and a team of volunteer editors compiled an electronic "anthology of protest." On March 5, a group gathered in Washington to symbolically present thirteen thousand poems by eleven thousand poets to the White House and Congress. Newspapers across the country covered the story of the cancelled symposium, the e-mailed poems, and the national days of poetry and protest held in more than two hundred cities and towns. At many of these events, writers read poems by or with reference to Hughes, Whitman, and Dickinson.

In Manchester, Vermont, on February 16, 2003, seven hundred people attended a "Poetry Reading in Honor of the Right to Protest as a Patriotic and Historical Tradition."[13] Julia Alvarez read "The White House Has Disinvited the Poets," excerpted below.

> Were they afraid the poets might persuade
> a sensitive girl who always loved to read,
> a librarian who stocked the shelves with Poe
> and Dickinson? . . .
> . . . .
> So why be afraid of us, Mrs. Bush? . . .
> We bring you the tidings of great joy—
> not only peace but poetry on earth.[14]

This gathering and others like it appear to answer the call of "POETLINE," written by San Francisco street poet Dennis Omowale Cutten in the 1990s.

> This is an emergency!
> I've an emergency!
> Are you there?
>
> I'm calling all poets . . .
> all poets . . .
> am calling all poets . . .
>   . . . can you hear me?!
>
> Damn! I thought I'd never
> get an answer.
> Now please listen:
>
> We must unite.
> Somehow, we've got
> to make good more
> appealing than evil.[15]

At the Vermont gathering, Ruth Stone began the evening with Dickinson's classic poem on humility, "I'm Nobody! Who are you?" Galway Kinnell read a poem that speaks for so many of us who fear that our leaders refuse to distinguish between good and evil, right and wrong.

> Much Madness is divinest Sense —
> To a discerning Eye —
> Much Sense — the starkest
> Madness —
> 'Tis the Majority
> In this — as all — prevail —
> Assent — and you are sane —
> Demur — you're straightway dangerous —
> And handled with a chain —

The poem's opening long line sets out a maxim. Short, divided lines, 3 and 4, create suspension ("starkest / Madness") and "Madness," dropped onto a line by itself, reverberates eerily. "Majority" alliterates with "Madness," an unsettling link, emphasizing that the majority wields the power to establish the authoritative definition of sanity. The rhyme of "sane" and "chain" once bothered me, because it seemed too easy, too perfect and pat. Then I started thinking, maybe that's the point—the majority wants to root out irregularity, difference, demurral, preventing a delay that would allow scruples to creep in. The rhyme and the poem's closure are paired jarringly with the open-endedness of the unrhymed first four lines, which resonate with foreboding.

In a matter of days after September 11, the political climate had shifted away from a time when Lynda Barry's Marlys and Maybonne could count peace signs among their "right ons" (favorite things), at the same time freely wrapping themselves together in the Stars and Stripes. Suddenly peace and protest were not patriotic, and saying they were could make you "straightway dangerous." Suddenly it was necessary for writer Barbara Kingsolver to invoke the national anthem and tell readers of her article "And Our Flag Was Still There" that "I would like to stand up for my flag and wave it over a few things I believe in, including but not limited to the protection of dissenting points of view."[16]

Later, a sign in front of the Unitarian Universalist meeting house in the center of Amherst, around the corner from the Emily Dickinson Museum, would feature a line from children's rights advocate and political theorist Marian Wright Edelman: "Democracy is not a spectator sport." Democracy cannot exist without responsible, engaged citizens debating complex national issues. "Much Madness is divinest Sense" serves as a touchstone for defending the right to dissent. During a 1986 conference for the centennial of Dickinson's death, held at the Folger Shakespeare Library in Washington, D.C., I heard Dickinson biographer Richard Sewall quote those lines and proclaim that they should be emblazoned on the dome of the U.S. Capitol.

Now, in political times such as these, when civil liberties are threatened and the right to dissent compromised, we remember that poetry can be a tool of democracy, adding to our understanding of history, helping us to access what we know, and leading us to examine our conscience. Dickinson's work belongs to a "poetry of illumination," as defined by Audre Lorde in her essay "Poetry Is Not a Luxury": "The quality of light by which we scrutinize our lives has direct bearing upon the product which we live, and upon the changes which we hope to bring about through those lives."[17] The hope provided by the light of Dickinson's poems may be the kind of hope described by the late twentieth-century Czech writer and political leader Václav Havel, who defines it as "not the conviction that something will turn out well, but the certainty that something makes sense regardless of how it turns out."[18]

REVOLUTION IS THE POD

On the day of poetry and protest in San Jose, California, at a noon reading downtown in Cesar Chavez Park, I read a Dickinson poem that I had first encountered thirty years earlier at the end of the war in Vietnam. A political activist from Canada whom I met on a tour of the Dickinson Homestead pointed this poem out to me as one that had inspired him.

> Revolution is the Pod
> Systems rattle from
> When the Winds of
> Will are stirred
> Excellent is Bloom
>
> But Except its' Russet
> Base
> Every Summer be
> The Entomber of itself,
> So of Liberty —
>
> Left inactive on the
> Stalk
> All its Purple fled
> Revolution shakes it
> for
> Test if it be dead —

I am moved by the poem's argument that seasonal cycles bear witness to the inevitability of change and by its view of the possibility that "Winds of / Will"— human will and, perhaps, divine will combined—can speed up a turnaround in a social hierarchy and restore a balance of power. Typical of Dickinson, the poem has both gravity and lightheartedness. "Revolution," a large, abstract concept, a four-syllable word, is equated with the little, monosyllabic "Pod." "Rattle" is a sound that could be playful or alarming, that could derive from something dead or alive. Bones? A musical instrument? A baby's toy? The warning of a snake about to strike? A death rattle in the breath? Possibilities of both life and death are evoked by the sound. Yet the rattle materializes as seeds. In nature, a seedcase bursts, seeds break out, new life emerges. In human systems, when something stops growing and changing, human and divine agency have to intervene to free the living from the dead. Bloom, new life, takes time but can be speeded up: "Excellent" puns on "excel" and "accelerate," high quality and increased speed. Renewal through the life cycle depends on roots, the russet base. Colors refer to clothing of the rulers and the ruled—the russet, reddish brown clothing of peasants and workers, the purple robes of royalty. At the end of the poem—"Revolution shakes it / for / Test if it be dead"—two lines teeter on "for." A new way of life hangs in the balance. For some people the political approach the poem advocates would be too conservative and too slow: keeping the roots and working within the system. For me, Dickinson's allegory captures a model of change that seems realistic, something that could be accomplished in time. I believe that human power and human creation, including poetry, can shake up the system and hasten the bloom of ideas.

A little Madness in the Spring

In the spring of 2004, the Emily Dickinson Museum conducted a week of activities honoring the museum's first full season of operation and celebrating National Poetry Month. The "Celebration of History and Poetry," "A little Madness in the Spring," included "A Community Marathon Reading of Emily Dickinson's Poems." For the first time the Homestead hosted a marathon-style reading of the 1,789 poems in Ralph Franklin's *Poems of Emily Dickinson*.

Six months later, in the preface to a report by the National Endowment for the Arts titled "Reading at Risk: A Survey of Literary Reading in America," poet Dana Gioia presented a "bleak assessment of the decline of reading's role in the nation's culture," stating that "for the first time in modern history, less than half of the adult population now reads literature."[19] One of the most comprehensive polls of art and literature consumption ever conducted, the report was based on twenty years of polling by the U.S. Census Bureau and used a sample of more than seventeen thousand adults. Literature is defined in this instance as novels, short stories, poems, and plays. Participants in the study were asked about the reading they did during leisure time, not at school or work. For every demographic category assessed—race, gender, age, income, educational level, region of the country—it was found that reading had declined. Overall, the reading of books of any kind has decreased, although not at the same rate as the reading of literature. The executive summary concludes, "If one believes that active and engaged readers lead richer intellectual lives than nonreaders and that a well-read citizenry is essential to a vibrant democracy, the decline of literary reading calls for serious action." [20]

The community reading of Dickinson's poems was spread over four days, lasting for twenty-seven hours and involving nearly as many groups of readers from the Amherst area and beyond. The poems were divided into sections of about sixty-five, and each hour was assigned to a specific group of people, usually eight to ten, who read the work in numerical, chronological order while sitting in a semicircle and facing an audience that varied in size throughout the day. Readers earned I READ A POEM buttons at the end of their hour. Participants represented a diverse range of organizations, including a Dickinson study group, a writing group, Learning in Retirement, the New Directions School, the Amherst Woman's Club, the Jones Library of Amherst, the National Yiddish Book Center, the Eric Carle Museum of Picture Book Art, and students, faculty, staff, and alumni from the five colleges (Amherst, Hampshire, Mount Holyoke, Smith, and the University of Massachusetts). At the end of each hour, audience members were invited to add their voices.

One group that came especially prepared was a class of fourth graders from the Cambridge Friends School. Students read their block of poems, many reciting stanzas from memory. Museum staff and guides began the reading, with codirector Jane Wald reading the first poem; Daria D'Arienzo, with Amherst College Archives and Special Collections, where so many of the manuscript poems reside, read the one thousandth poem (by chance!), and I had the honor of reading the last poem as Emily Dickinson International Society members took the final hour.

Beautifully organized, and highlighting the power of Dickinson's appeal as well as the chemistry that develops among people as they read poetry out loud and to each other, the marathon was exciting, demanding, and revealing—awesome in the Dickinsonian as well as the currently popular sense of the word. In a set of instructions mailed out to participants, museum codirector Cindy Dickinson noted, "It will be an adventure!" It was.

A little
Madness in
the Spring
Is wholesome
Even for the
King —
But God be
with the Clown —

Who ponders
this tremendous
scene,
This whole
Experiment of
Green,
As if it
were his own!

The madness of spring and the madness of a marathon are playful, joyful kinds of madness. Yet participants at the community reading were seriously engaged as they read; one organization after another took its place in the circle of chairs and became absorbed in the poetry as if settling into a study group. One of my favorite moments was when a young woman's turn came to read and she sat studying the page. "Oh," she said, when she looked up and saw us waiting for her, "I was still thinking about the last poem."

We know, to borrow Lorde's words, that "poetry is not a luxury." Galway Kinnell calls "Much Madness is divinest Sense" a "perception and warning."[21] To an extent, the same can be said of "A little Madness in the Spring." Don't be arrogant, the poem warns. Don't act like you own everything. Life is an experiment, and it's uncertain. The verb "ponder" is important in this poem, which points out that thinking, even well-intentioned thought, can lead to self-deception. The king needs humility. If he acts like a clown, a foolish person, if his kingly pride overtakes him, if he starts to believe that he will rule the world forever, he's in danger. And so, too, is the world. "Whole"—the poem uses both "whole" and "wholesome"—derives from "hale," which means healthy. In a poem that begins, "A Counterfeit — / a Plated Person — / I would not be" (J1453/Fr1514), Dickinson defines truth as "good Health — and Safety, and the Sky." "A little Madness in the Spring" urges me not to give in to the delusion of power, whether my "king" side or my "clown" side is out to mislead me. Truth, health, just a little madness—these are the guideposts Dickinson sets out. Through protest readings and community readings, e-mail and bulletin boards, newsletters and comic strips, museums and libraries, classrooms and literary societies—may the circle of Dickinson readers be unbroken.

NOTES

1. The text of the Dickinson poems in this essay are edited print translations, the work of the author. Poem reference numbers for the standard editions, and page numbers for the manuscript books, are as follows: "The Poets light but Lamps" (J883/Fr930/MB1065); "After great pain, a formal feeling comes" (J341/Fr372/MB395); "Much Madness is divinest Sense" (J435/Fr620/MB680); "Revolution is the Pod" (J1082/Fr1044/MB1253); "A little Madness in the Spring" (J1333/Fr1356).

2. The Emily Dickinson Museum includes the Homestead, home of the poet, and the Evergreens, home of the poet's brother and sister-in-law. See www.emilydickinsonmuseum.org for the complete text of the mission statement.

3. Dinitia Smith, "In Shelley or Auden, in the Sonnet or Free Verse, the Eerily Intimate Power of Poetry to Console," *New York Times,* October 1, 2001.

4. W. H. Auden, "September 1, 1939," in *Staying Alive: Real Poems for Unreal Times,* ed. Neil Astley (New York: Miramax/Hyperion, 2003), 356–58.

5. Margo Jefferson, "The News from Poetry," *New York Times Book Review,* May 11, 2003.

6. Neil Astley, ed., *Staying Alive: Real Poems for Unreal Times* (New York: Miramax/Hyperion, 2003), 356–58. *Staying Alive* was published in 2002 in Great Britain by Bloodaxe Books. The lines from Dickinson and Kafka appear on the unnumbered page preceding the title page. Dickinson's remarks were made to Thomas Higginson, who recorded them for his wife in a letter written on August 16, 1870, presumably the date of their conversation. See Johnson, Letter 342a.

7. Ibid., 26.

8. The Homestead advisory committee predated the Emily Dickinson Museum.

9. The quotations here are from an e-mail that Hamill began to circulate on January 19, 2003.

10. Noelia Rodriguez, spokeswoman for Laura Bush, gave this explanation on January 29, 2003, when the cancellation of the White House symposium was first announced. Rodriguez's statement was widely quoted by the press.

11. Robert Pinsky, "Statement of Conscience," in *Poets Against the War,* ed. Sam Hamill, with Sally Anderson et al. (New York: Thunder's Mouth Press/Nation Books, 2003), 180–81.

12. See http://www.poetsagainstthewar.org and Hamill's "New Year's Letter 2004."

13. Proceedings of this event, poems, and prefatory remarks by poets and organizers are presented in *Cry Out: Poets Protest the War* (New York: George Braziller, 2003).

14. Julia Alvarez, "The White House Has Disinvited the Poets," in *Cry Out,* 87.

15. "POETLINE" was published in the fall 2003 special poetry issue of the Bay Area "street sheet," *Street Spirit,* sponsored by the Friends Service Committee. Donations support the homeless. A note to the poem explains that in the late 1990s Cutten died of a brain tumor.

16. Barbara Kingsolver, "And Our Flag Was Still There," *San Francisco Chronicle,* September 25, 2001.

17. Audre Lorde, "Poetry Is Not a Luxury," in *Sister Outsider: Essays and Speeches* (Trumansburg, N.Y.: Crossing Press, 1984), 36.

18. Havel is quoted by Margaret Wheatley in her essay "From Hope to Hopelessness," in *The Impossible Will Take a Little While: A Citizen's Guide to Hope in a Time of Fear,* ed. Paul Rogat Loeb (New York: Basic Books, 2004), 349. Loeb's collection takes its title from the Army Core of Engineers motto during World War II: "The difficult I'll do right now. The impossible will take a little while" (4).

19. Dana Gioia, "Reading at Risk: A Survey of Literary Reading in America," National Endowment for the Arts, Research Division Report 46, June 2004, vii. The report is available online at the NEA Web site: www.arts.gov.

20. Ibid., ix.

21. Galway Kinnell, "To the States, to Identify . . . ," in *Cry Out,* 52.

Emily Dickinson
The Other That I Am

MARION WOODMAN

I grew up in small Ontario towns with fresh morning air, lush green lawns, cascading flower gardens, several splendid houses, and several well-attended churches; I called one of these small churches home, and in its pastoral environment I was raised with my two younger brothers. Throughout our childhood, we were rarely far from each other. Our father, a minister, was a beloved pastor to his congregation. Our mother was stricken with tuberculosis when I was four; nevertheless, she fought to live, and did, until she was seventy-five. I silently watched her struggle, knowing that any disturbance would not contribute to the harmony necessary for her survival. The strong maternal container that would have delighted in her daughter's coming into her own womanhood was not there. Moreover, the graveyard was not far from the parsonage; it was in my cells.

One of my preschool delights was taking my doll to the graveyard for a reading lesson. There I kept my own little dishes under a log just in case someone needed tea. If a parishioner had come to visit the grave of a loved one, I always eyed the beautiful flowers before they were placed on the grave. My tea table—a large, flat, granite slab with REBECCA chiseled into it—needed bright colors. Leaving my doll to guard the dishes, I went to listen to the story. I listened, asked questions, and when the moment seemed right, I invited the brokenhearted to come for tea and bring a flower. These encounters did not seem strange to me or to my guests, who recounted their stories, detail by detail, to me and my doll.

This is my story. Reading it now, I am once again struck by similar details in Emily Dickinson's story. Our childhoods were mostly lived in the spaceless, timeless world of the imagination—the eternal world that one enters through ritual. Death was just on the other side of the gate. In our family, we three children almost always played marriage, baptism, or funeral. I often accompanied my father

All citations of Dickinson's poems used in this chapter are from *The Poems of Emily Dickinson,* ed. Thomas H. Johnson, 3 vols. (Cambridge, Mass.: Harvard Univ. Press, 1955).

on his visits of solace to the families who had received messages from overseas that their sons or fathers had been killed or were missing in action. Here was the seedbed of my love for Emily Dickinson, rooted in archetypal patterns.

When I was perhaps nine years old, I was very ill with whooping cough. Gray-haired Maggi came to the kitchen door to return our family laundry that she, good neighbor that she was, had washed and ironed. With it was a little red book entitled *Poems of Emily Dickinson* and a handwritten greeting, "From the Neighbor Women on the Corner." Delighted with my new book, I instantly plunged into it and found the friend I had so long yearned for, someone who didn't turn away from pain and the graveyard gate. From that day until this, I have increasingly been aware of our kinship. In knowing her poetry at an ever-deepening level, I realize how our subterranean corridors were mirrored in a shared imagery and how I recognized myself there, both through similarity and nonsimilarity, as the Other that I am.

That soul connection deepens as the threads of my life are being woven into a completed tapestry. I can connect with Emily anytime, anywhere, through a line, through a word, through a metaphor. My love of language began when I was three and my father taught me to sound *a*'s and *o*'s, discovering worlds within letters. As he hoed his roses, I read to him from my primer. Now I sound to myself as I memorize poetry on an airplane.

The Moments of Dominion
That happen on the Soul
And leave it with a Discontent
Too exquisite — to tell — (J627/Fr696)

Another world was in the church into which I could slip any afternoon and wait for God. It was a complete mystery that my father said God was there, but I could neither see nor hear Him. Finally, however, I did understand words like "mystery," "Eternity," "Angels," "Presence," "Calvary," and "Resurrection." I did not delight in Mary, John, and Peter, the characters in my primer, when I went to school.

Death and life were juxtaposed—the movement from life in this world to immortality was a mere adjustment in focus. Immortality was not death, but a sense of Presence, an intersection between eternal and transitory. This archetypal Presence was and is still the foundation of my life.

Unfortunately, or fortunately, preachers' kids are not part of the social structure of a school insofar as they are outsiders. Because the family moves every four or five years, the kids are constantly coping with new acquaintances, incongruous school timetables, parents who are trying to sail with the crosscurrents in a new congregation. Expectations of goodness, faith, honesty, brilliance are loaded onto these waifs of fortune by adult parishioners; curiosity, jealousy, fear drift around them from their peers.

The world in which I lived until the age of thirteen was a world of trance. I did not do well at school. I played the piano well. I kept scores for the athletes. My wide-open blue eyes and silent tongue masked the intensity of my search, the violence of my feelings, the ferocity of my rebellion. At school, I was a good girl, a quiet, gentle listener. At home, I rocked in the big rocking chair in my room, reading my beloved friend's poetry as loudly as I wished. Downstairs my father was often reading Robbie Burns in a similar manner, for a similar reason. Certainly the intensity of my passion, the intensity of my budding sexuality, the intensity of my yearning for something beyond what the world provides—all were in that rocking. In my aloneness, even God was against me.

> Of Course — I prayed —
> And did God Care?
> He cared as much as on the Air
> A Bird — had stamped her foot —
> And cried "Give Me" —
> My Reason — Life —
> I had not had — but for Yourself —
> 'Twere better Charity
> To leave me in the Atom's Tomb —
> Merry, and Nought, and gay, and numb —
> Than this smart Misery. (J376/Fr581)

Throughout high school, I never heard of therapy, or trauma, or psychology. Nor was there any such thing in the towns where I lived. Knowing that another young girl, young Emily, wrote the words that I dared not think opened all the repressions and depressions of my young life. My faith in God was a child's faith; my idealistic hopes were not met. God was my Assailant. I had no one to turn to, no container to contain either my rage or my grief—no one but Emily Dickinson. I too was seriously asking myself, "Could it be Madness — this?" (J410/Fr423).

Gradually, I recognized the fun-loving, high-spirited young woman inside of me who was determined to break out of her prison.

Our lives are Swiss —
So still — so Cool —
Till some odd afternoon
The Alps neglect their Curtains
And we look farther on!

Italy stands the other side!
While like a guard between
The solemn Alps —
The siren Alps
Forever intervene! (J80/Fr129)

Yes, I eventually fell in love, and yes, the divine projection without a human receptor deeply wounded me. From where I now stand, with years of my life behind me, I can say this was the first and, therefore, my profoundest descent into the underworld. In a similar situation, Emily Dickinson wrote at least a poem a day for one year "To hold [her] Senses — on" (J443/Fr522). Because I had come to know her so well, I knew if I were going to save my sanity, I had to write in my journal daily and read at least one of her poems aloud. Not all of them were focused on pain. Each encounter with a friend, flower, bird, or bee released bolts of energy that were transformed into original images. Knowing that Emily was able to hold some kind of balance enabled me to be aware enough to participate in life while bringing to consciousness the content of my projection, pulling back its energy into myself, and finding new creative outlets, new containers, for its strength.[1]

Such a projection comes from the divine energy of a father-god complex. When that father arrow is released, it carries the energy of the unconscious God for whom I waited many a childhood afternoon in my father's church. Not only the father, but everything the father represents in the culture—education, church, law, institutions—will unconsciously be activated. The all-loving God is also the all-powerful God that demands the woman's obedience to, or her rebellion against, such a dictator. A projection is let loose from the unconscious like an arrow. The man or woman it hits becomes the magnet that controls her soul. Around the beloved she fantasizes an ideal world in which she is loved, more often rejected. Empowered in a fantasy that can never be realized, she splits her secret world off from the outer world. She is left with willpower and a mask to cover a blistering wound.

Reading Emily's poetry allowed me to drop into my own depths to bring to consciousness what I was feeling and acting out. Her genius for holding the tensions of the opposites made me recognize the anguish that was orchestrated more fiercely within the dashes and capitals than what spoke between them. She taught me how to hold a "bomb in my bosom" and remain calm. Only later was I able to endure the "bolts" that demanded maturity and a deeper understanding of my body's need for expression. My Self knew then and knows now the danger of depression if passion and reason are separated. Authenticity demands that body and soul speak together.

Well, I've been around a few sharp curves in the journey since I pulled myself out of that maelstrom. "Pulling myself out" means pulling back into myself the energy that I unconsciously sent into or onto other people, thus giving away my power, my creativity, even my faith. Taking responsibility for my projections is the Jungian way of describing this most painful task of growing up. Taking responsibility for my shadow projections was part of that labor.

Through an intimate knowledge of Dickinson's poetry, I was able, line by line, to understand the surrendering of my ego desires—desires that could never be fulfilled—and realign my faith to what God desired. This has been a lifetime process—moving from being a victim to stepping into my own destiny, claiming the authenticity of my own life.

Emily Dickinson opened the floodgates that released my grief and rebellion into delight in the broader Circumference. She gave meaning to my imagery. She gave me exquisite language to differentiate my deepest hunches, horrors, hopes, and intuitions. She gave me a transformer right at the center of my Being that had sufficient voltage to change destruction into creation. My own creativity now reverberates in my life, keeping my soul open and my spirit fiery. She returned to me the life-giving garden I had treasured as a child, Nature in her glory as Goddess of the tiniest and mightiest.

> When "Landlords" turn the drunken Bee
> Out of the Foxglove's door —
> When Butterflies — renounce their "drams" —
> I shall but drink the more! . . . (J214/Fr207)

Emily Dickinson was able to hold that precious edge that released her own dancing star, that star that was her mature Being. She learned not to look too far ahead or too far behind. Now is enough. I open her poems—a dazzling metaphor dances out to me.

> Narcotics cannot still the Tooth
> That nibbles at the soul. . . . (J501/Fr373)

NOTE

1. I have written about the anguish of redeeming this projection in *Addiction to Perfection: The Still Unravished Bride; A Psychological Study* (Toronto: Inner City Books, 1982) and *The Pregnant Virgin: A Process of Psychological Transformation* (Toronto: Inner City Books, 1985). I discussed on audiotape the transformative powers of Emily Dickinson's poetry in *Emily Dickinson and the Demon Lover* (Boulder, Colo.: Sounds True, 1993).

Poetry is what in a poem makes you laugh, cry, prickle, be silent, makes your toe nails twinkle, makes you want to do this or that or nothing, makes you know that you are not alone in the unknown world, that your bliss and suffering is forever shared and forever all your own.

DYLAN THOMAS

Emily Dickinson! How does one tackle that subject!? She's mystical, lyrical, and astonishing! She can evoke ecstasy—as in "Bring me the sunset in a cup." Makes you want to dance and sing! She can make you giggle—"The Grass so little has to do." Puts you in a laughing mood! She can stop your breath and rearrange your thinking about a subject you though *only* you were privy to.

ANNE JACKSON, ACTOR
Jackson is known for her lively readings of Emily Dickinson's poetry.

"Will there really be a 'morning'?"

A Lamp on the Journey through Pain

BARBARA DANA

> The Poets light but Lamps —
> Themselves — go out —
> The Wicks they stimulate
> If vital Light
>
> Inhere as do the Suns —
> Each Age a Lens
> Disseminating their
> Circumference — (J883/Fr930)

I am in need of consolation. Two dear friends have just died—dearest of the dear!—one, three days ago, on my birthday. How could he have died on my birthday? How could he have been so careless? Maybe he wasn't being careless. Maybe it was his way of being close, of resting where he felt secure. Maybe it was a message that he was thinking of me. Maybe it meant he never wanted me to forget him—as if that were possible. Maybe it meant nothing. "But, what of that?" (J301/Fr403)

I see his birthday presents on the table, bought two months ago, eagerness having its way with me. Etude—Pinot Noir—2003. His favorite. And a tiny model of Brahms made in Germany. He loved Germany. And Brahms. He was conducting Brahms when we met—familiar beyond familiar. When I first saw him it had been like coming home. I knew him completely. The way he picked up the chair, the way he held his hand against his belt, fingers curved, knuckles high. The strength, the sensitivity, the pain, the joy, alive at once in that hand!

All citations of Dickinson's poems used in this chapter are from *The Poems of Emily Dickinson,* ed. R. W. Franklin, 3 vols. (Cambridge, Mass.: Harvard Univ. Press, 1998).

Long Years apart — can make no
Breach a second cannot fill —
The absence of the Witch does not
Invalidate the spell —

The embers of a Thousand Years
Uncovered by the Hand
That fondled them when they were Fire
Will stir and understand (J1383/Fr1405)

How do I live without him?

I want to tell my dog. I want to bury my face in his warm black coat and tell him how hard this is, to rest in his steady acceptance and love. But he is the other friend that died, gone last month. Jesse, my "Shaggy Ally" (L280), my Carlo, my constant companion for fifteen years. German shepherds don't usually live that long. Newfoundlands like Emily's Carlo don't often live to be sixteen either. I remember a letter Emily wrote to Thomas Wentworth Higginson when Carlo died. I look it up.

Carlo died —
     E. Dickinson
     Would you instruct me now? (L314)

The spare despair! She knows! "Pain — has an Element of Blank" (J650/Fr760). I feel that blankness now.

I *know* that Emily knows what I am feeling. I feel her with me, no separation, no waiting until I come to my senses. I am *at* my senses. No beating about the bush, no pretending. She appreciates that. "I like a look of Agony, / Because I know it's true" (J241/Fr339).

Emily's words run through my mind as I write today, thought after thought tumbling end over end.

My first well Day — since many ill —
I asked to go abroad,
And take the Sunshine in my hands
And see the things in Pod— (J574/Fr288)

I gave that poem to my friend when his mother died and he had been going through a period of grieving. He told me that the poem had comforted him and inspired him too. He put the final stanza on his refrigerator.

My loss, by sickness — Was it Loss?
Or that Ethereal Gain
One earns by measuring the Grave —
Then — measuring the Sun —

I brought him other of Emily's poems in the hospital and cards with her razor-light messages to cut through the morass of pain. I wanted so badly to make everything better, to bring him that thing that would make the difference, that would take away the possibility of his dying, but I couldn't think of what it was. The last card I brought him came from the Homestead in Amherst, where Emily was born and lived and died. The card had butterflies on it, all purple and yellow with hope. Underneath the butterflies it said, "I told my Soul to sing" (J410/Fr423). I knew it was for him. Inside the card I copied, in shaky letters, the only thing I could think to bring him.

It's all I have to bring today —
This, and my heart beside —
This, and my heart, and all the fields —
And all the meadows wide —
Be sure you count — sh'd I forget
Some one the sum could tell —
This, and my heart, and all the Bees
Which in the Clover dwell. (J26/Fr17)

He read it quietly and long. When he finished reading he paused, looking over the top of the card in the direction of the doorframe, or the clock above the nurses' station in the hall, not seeing those things, it seemed. And at last, "Thank you," he said. In my shyness, Emily had spoken for me and comforted us both.

The loss of my beloved friend is unacceptable and yet somehow I must accept it, as I must accept the loss of my dog. I need help. I must remember how Emily was there with me before and ask her to help me now. If that sounds overly personal, it is. That's what my relationship with Emily has been. I think that's what makes it work.

. . .

Several years ago when my marriage ended and my father died in the same winter I didn't know much about Emily Dickinson. I had seen Julie Harris play Emily some twenty-five years before in William Luce's play *The Belle of Amherst* and had been moved by Julie's radiant performance. I am both an actor and a writer and in those days was concentrating on my acting. That being the case, Julie's masterful work was what captivated me most of all. I marveled at the spirit and spunk of the woman she played but somehow did not immediately pursue a further connection to the poet. That would come later.

"Later" was a dark time. Thirty-five-year marriage—over. Beloved father—dead. My cousin had just died too, my cousin who was like a brother—two only children, bonded since childhood. He was a jazz musician. Cancer of the esophagus. It had been an awful death. It was all too much.

The worst thing about that time was waking up in the morning. That terrible moment of remembering! Check the clock. Five thirty. It's early. And then—Oh, God. My husband is gone. My father is dead. My "brother" is dead. My life is over—I forgot! The numbness, the squeeze in the heart, the sinking down to a place of nothing. "There is a pain — so utter — / It swallows substance up" (J599/Fr515).

I used to wish I could think about the unthinkable every second so that I could avoid the awful moment of remembering the "Funeral, in my Brain" (J280/Fr340). Lying in bed in the semidarkness, sleepless, I wondered, Why get up? I couldn't figure it out. "And then a Plank in Reason, broke, / And I dropped down, and down" (J280/Fr340).

I have the dubious luxury of being a freelance artist. At the time, I had no acting job, no writing deadline. I used to think it would be easier if I had a "real" job, the kind I had to show up for or be fired from. It might have gotten me out of the house. But there I lay, wondering. Should I do something? Take a shower, perhaps? Why? I would just get dirty again and have to take another shower tomorrow. Make my bed? I would just mess it up when I got back into it, tired from a day of doing things. What things? My mind was blank. There used to be things. I figured I could save a lot of trouble and energy by lying still. I could wait for death, ultimate, total, and complete. Not so different from right now, but simpler, easier to understand. Then I would think of Jesse. I had to walk him, but I was too exhausted to move.

One of my daughters-in-law prepared her morning coffee at night so that when she got up it was ready to go. I had taken the cue from her and had begun setting up the coffee before I went to bed. My morning had a goal. Get from the bed to the coffee machine. I could handle that. One step at a time.

Steps were hard, though. My legs were weak, giving way without notice, and I often had trouble breathing. I couldn't seem to breathe below my neck. I would get faint and have to sit down or, better yet, lie down. I alarmed myself one night when I got up to go to the bathroom and saw my reflection in the mirror. I was wearing a neck brace for a pinched nerve, a splint on each wrist for carpel tunnel syndrome, and a mouth guard because I was grinding my teeth in my sleep. Quite a vision!

Each morning after walking Jesse I would head for the gray couch with the torn slipcover in the living room. I was too exhausted for anything besides a nap. My eyes usually fell on my CD collection, directly in my line of vision as my head rested on the soft, colorful cushion my ex-husband and I had purchased at the suggestion of the interior designer who lived down the street from us in Chappaqua in the days when I had a life. I used to love music, but I couldn't listen to it anymore. Music enjoyed in happy times was too painful now that the happy times were gone. Sad music put me over the edge. I thought I should get some new music, but I couldn't think of what. And even if I could think of something to buy, there would be the horror of the panic attack I was sure to have in the parking lot before even reaching the store.

The best thing about that time was that my son, Matthew, and his wife, Pamela, were staying with me. They had been living in California when Matthew got a part in a play on Broadway and were now living with me until they could get settled on the East Coast. Pamela was pregnant with my grandson, Sam. Pamela had been directing in Los Angeles and wanted to direct me in something off-Broadway. She wanted me to play Emily Dickinson in *The Belle of Amherst*. I told her there was no way I would consider that. It had been done perfectly by Julie Harris and I wouldn't presume to even think about it. We had taken to reading plays once a week, a joy for her and a kind of therapy for me, upstairs in my study over the garage. One day Pamela suggested we read *The Belle of Amherst*. When I reminded her that there was only one role in the play, she told me it didn't matter. She wanted to hear it. She would read the stage directions. For some reason, I agreed. I felt removed, not present, blank, as I had been feeling for months.

After great pain, a formal feeling comes —
The Nerves sit ceremonious, like Tombs —
The stiff Hear questions "was it He, that bore,"
And "Yesterday, or Centuries before"?

The Feet, mechanical, go round —
A Wooden way
Of Ground, or Air, or Ought —
Regardless grown,
A Quartz contentment, like a stone —

This is the Hour of Lead —
Remembered, if outlived,

As Freezing persons, recollect the Snow —
First — Chill — then Stupor — then the letting go — (J341/Fr372)

As Emily, I read. "When the Best is gone—I know that other things are not of consequence—The Heart wants what it wants—or else it does not care" (L262). My nose begins to itch and I realize I am about to cry. I continue as Emily, reciting a poem.

Will there really be a "morning"?
Is there such a thing as "Day"?
Could I see it from the mountains
If I were as tall as they?

Has it feet like Water lilies?
Has it feathers like a Bird?
Is it brought from famous countries
Of which I have never heard?

Oh some Scholar! Oh some Sailor!
Oh some Wise Man from the skies!
Please to tell a little Pilgrim
Where the place called "morning" lies! (J101/Fr148)

I broke apart. It was a jolt out of the blankness of despair. A crack, a split! Not only heart but chest as well and stomach split apart. And all at once tears and great sobbing, as if truth had finally come home. The pain but also the glorious feeling of aliveness. This is true! This is how I am! This is *real*! And someone knows. I am not alone!

I think I cried most of the way through the reading. When we were done I knew I had to be close to this woman. I had to know her, to keep her with me so that I would be all right. The way I chose to do that was not to *act* her, as one might have expected, but to call my editor at HarperCollins and suggest that I write a book about her. I had written a historical novel based on the young life of Joan of Arc for Harpers, and they had been after me to write a novel based on the early life of some other strong woman. I wasn't interested. I had done that. Who could be more exciting than Joan? That had been my feeling, but not anymore. I got a contract and began my work, an extraordinary journey of artistic fulfillment and personal healing.

Julie Harris has recorded an incredible two-tape set of readings of Emily's poems and letters. I lived with these tapes, becoming Emily so I that I could write about her. I began walking, slowly at first, headphones in place, tape player in my jacket pocket, walking and crying and beginning to live again.

Several poems hit me especially hard. One day as I pass the graveyard next to the church across the street from my new "alone house" in South Salem, my companion, Emily, speaks to me, knowing where I am and there with me.

> Heart! We will forget him!
> You and I — tonight!
> You may forget the warmth he gave —
> I will forget the light!
>
> When you have done, pray tell me
> That I may straight begin!
> Haste! lest while you're lagging
> I remember him! (J47/Fr64)

I gasp. I sob. I hold my heart. Another day I pass the antique store next to the deli on my way back from a walk around the lake. It's starting to rain. Emily's voice is in my ears.

> I cautious, scanned my little life —
> I winnowed what would fade
> From what w'd last till Heads like mine
> Should be a'dreaming laid.
>
> I put the latter in a Barn —
> The former, blew away.
> I went one winter morning
> And lo, my priceless Hay
>
> Was not upon the "Scaffold" —
> Was not upon the "Beam" —
> And from a thriving Farmer —
> A Cynic, I became.
>
> Whether a Thief did it —
> Whether it was the wind —
> Whether Deity's guiltless —
> My business is, to find!

So I begin to ransack!
How is it Hearts, with Thee?
Art thou within the little Barn
Love provided Thee? (J178/Fr175)

I sit on the stone wall that borders the graveyard across the street from the deli.
I take off my headphones and cry for awhile. I think this poem hit me hardest
of all. Emily knew me. She saw what I was going through. She would be the
lamp on my journey through pain.

I have never found another way to deal with pain other than to go through
it. I have found this to be true in therapy and, as with Emily, have welcomed
the wise and compassionate presence of my therapist. When going through a
difficult time, I feel that if I can't avoid the pain I will surely die. I feel that the
pain will always be there. "It has no Future — but itself — / Its Infinite contain
/ Its Past — enlightened to perceive / New Periods — of Pain"(J650/Fr760).
I remember thinking when Emily helped me that first time that friends and
acquaintances were so caring, so supportive, but that they didn't know what I
was feeling. I thought if they really knew, they wouldn't say things like "Time
heals everything" and "You're stronger than you think." I heard about "moving
on" and "getting closure" and wondered what that meant. What was closure
anyway? I didn't want to close. I wanted to open! But I couldn't. I was all shut
down. Didn't they realize I was dying? For whatever reason, they couldn't make
it clear to me that they knew what I was going through, or I couldn't see it. I
needed to know they had been there.

Unto a broken heart
No other one may go
Without the high prerogative
Itself hath suffered too (J1704/Fr1745)

Emily's poems served me in many ways. First, they were maps: This is what
you're feeling now. Later you may feel this. Then this. And you will live. I sensed
the authenticity of her words. I knew she had been there. The originality and
specific immediacy of her message spoke to the child within me who, despite
the pain, longed to be told the truth. Yes, she told me, there is pain. It can be awful. And, yes, it will end. Most often it is not death. It only appears to be. That,
for me, was a crucial point because not knowing that the pain would end made
it unbearable to endure. It reminded me of the Lamaze classes I took when I

was pregnant with my son, Anthony. The thing I valued most about the classes was the message that a contraction would last for a certain amount of time and then it would end. There would be another and another, but there would be spaces between the contractions in which to rest. The baby would be born. The pain would end.

According to Emily, "The Province of the Saved" is "To qualify Despair / To Those who failing new — / Mistake Defeat for Death — Each time — / Till acclimated — to" (J539/Fr659). I read her words and feel acclimated. I think, if she can feel this much pain and survive, maybe I can too.

In Joan Didion's book *The Year of Magical Thinking*, she writes brilliantly about her personal experience of grief. I am with her, as I am with Emily. She is with me. I am strengthened by taking this journey with her. At one point Didion quotes Eric Lindemann, chief of psychiatry at Massachusetts General Hospital in the 1940s who interviewed family members of people killed in a fire in Coconut Grove in 1942. In the study, he defines the phenomenon of grief.[1] Like other valuable studies, his is a roadmap for what can be expected on the journey through the process of grieving, consoling on one level but not nearly as consoling for me as the rest of the book. A study takes me only so far. There is the possibility of ending up feeling awash in a sea of statistics. When one is grieving there is all too much danger of doubting one's existence. That's how it is for me. At times, all I can feel is the pain. I can't perceive *myself* there, feeling it. Identifying with Emily, which because of her particular genius is virtually impossible not to do, I see—*become*—an *individual* going through the process of grief. I'm not lost in the process. This makes it bearable. It seems to me that however difficult the process, I have my footing when standing in what's *real*. However painful, the "realness" brings me home to who I am and to the knowledge that I exist. Emily brings me home to the truth of my own soul. From there I can begin.

I have spent the last several years with Emily. I began walking with my tape player and listening to Julie Harris speak her words—walking, crying, feeling the joy of recognition and companionship, unable to separate my writing work from my personal journey of growth and healing. Each day I read—Emily's poetry and letters; Richard Sewall's biography and Alfred Habegger's; Polly Longsworth's vivid *The World of Emily Dickinson*; and essays, novels, and on and on.

That first summer after moving into my first "alone house," I couldn't shop or cook without encountering fearsome panic attacks, so each evening I gathered up whatever ED book I was reading and went to the little café two miles down on Route 35 for dinner—a glass of Pinot Grigio, broiled salmon, salad, and Emily. I was healing.

A sure sign of my healing process was when, in the midst of a panic attack in the parking lot of D'Agostino's market—heart pounding, knees giving way, unable to breathe—I nevertheless thought, I can use this in my book. Emily had panic attacks. Remember how it feels. It will make the book more true. As I witnessed my panic, I couldn't help but realize that I existed apart from the fear. I was witnessing it. That meant there was another part of me, besides the "me" that was caught in the fear. I think Emily and I helped each other in that moment. As she helped me through the panic, I helped her by getting to know her more deeply, thereby being more able to convey the truth of her in my work.

I spent a great deal of time in Amherst researching my book, standing in Emily's room, looking out her window, sitting in her parlor, walking her walk to school, to church, sitting under the oak tree in the garden she loved so well, watching her sunset. "But how he set — I know not — / There seemed a purple stile / That little Yellow boys and girls / Were climbing all the while" (J318/Fr204). I stood by her cradle in the hallway outside her room and at her grave a short distance away.

The first time I ventured on a road trip alone it was for research. I collected my Emily tapes and CDs, including my favorites, of course, by Julie Harris, and headed for the Homestead. I also packed the wonderful tape of Marion Woodman's *Emily Dickinson and the Demon Lover* along with my Sewall biography, my notebook, my edition of the collected poems, my edition of the letters, my pens, my pencils, my camera, my courage, and my sunhat. At the last minute I grabbed a surprising item, a CD entitled *The Greatest Hits of the Beach Boys*. My jazz musician cousin/"brother" had mentioned the Beach Boys a few months earlier in Los Angeles shortly before he died. We had been on our way to one of his radiation treatments. He wore a blue windbreaker and carried a shoebox filled with his medications to show to some doctor or other at the hospital. As we crossed Beverly Boulevard, he said, "Do you like the Beach Boys?" I told him I did but hadn't listened to them in a long time. "Great harmonies," he said. "The Beatles were influenced by them, you know." I hadn't known that and told him so. Later I bought the CD, but he died before I got a chance to listen to it and then I didn't want to. I hadn't been able to listen to music for months. Maybe on the way to Amherst, I thought.

It was May when I packed up my father's '88 Toyota Camry and headed north, leaving my beloved Jesse at home with his dog sitter because they didn't take dogs at the B&B. I was really alone but I didn't feel that way. Emily was with me. And as it turned out, so were the Beach Boys. After listening to Julie's tapes and to Marion Woodman's, I reached for the Beach Boys and put them on. It was a clear day—deep blue sky, no clouds, warm. I opened the driver's side window on Route 84 as the Beach Boys sang, "*Surf City, here we come. . . .*"

I actually felt joy.

Months later, when the Beach Boys gave a concert at the Palace Theatre in Stamford, Connecticut, I was moved to order a ticket. I knew the theater well. I had played Joan of Arc in a production of *Joan of Loraine* there when I was in my thirties. I went by myself, but Emily was in my purse. I carried her words with me wherever I went—bolts of lightning energy jogging my mind into feeling, like shock treatments, quotes that one puts on the refrigerator to bring oneself back into perspective.

> We never know how high we are
> Till we are called to rise
> And then if we are true to plan
> Our statures touch the skies — . . . (J1176/Fr1197)

These words were in my wallet. Sitting in my front row seat, I took them out and read them. I looked about the theater. I knew every exit door, every chandelier, every piece of molding. Never mind that it had been twenty years since I had been on that stage. I was home. The Beach Boys made their entrance. Applause. They started to play. And sing. I felt so good, so connected to myself and to everyone in the theater. I looked about the audience—parents with children, grandparents with grandchildren, middle-aged people, couples holding hands, students and artists, musicians and writers, bankers and lawyers, all into the music, into each other, into the day itself. Once again Emily's words echoed my own.

> To have been made alive is so chief a thing . . . (L860)

. . .

Tomorrow is my friend's birthday. His presents are still on the table by the window. I had planned to celebrate with him. Now I must find a way to celebrate without him. I will go to his grave and put some yellow roses on the spot where his ashes are buried. I bought the roses today because tomorrow is Sunday and I don't know whether I can buy flowers on Sunday.

It was good to remind myself of how Emily helped me through my last time of grief. It's been helpful, although a challenge, to write about the matter of healing pain while at the same time experiencing it. Emily could do it. She had the amazing ability to hold the most specific sensations of pain alive while containing the sensations in such a way as to make them endurable. Her ability to do this helps me so much. I wonder if it helped her too.

Tomorrow I will take the yellow roses to the graveyard beside the little church. I expect I will have many feelings there. I've been thinking a lot about death since I lost my friend. Where is he now? What is eternity? Does it even exist? I know there is more to life than we can see. "This World is not Conclusion" (J501/Fr373). But what does my friend think? *Is* he thinking?

Last week I listened to a poem of Emily's on my way to Amherst for a poetry discussion led by scholar and poet Joy Ladin. It was warm for January. Spring will be here soon, I thought. I was wondering about whether or not my friend knew how much I loved him. Did he know how much I had wanted to do something to keep him alive? I had tried, but I couldn't do it.

I passed the Common, turned right on Main Street, and headed for the Homestead as Emily's words sounded on the tape.

> If I should'nt be alive
> When the Robins come,
> Give the one in Red Cravat,
> A Memorial crumb —
>
> If I could'nt thank you,
> Being fast asleep,
> You will know I'm trying
> With my Granite lip! (J182/Fr210)

I looked up at Emily's window through tears.

· · ·

So. Tomorrow at the grave. I know what to expect, some of it anyway. Emily has already let me in on it.

> There is a finished feeling
> Experienced at Graves —
> A leisure of the Future —
> A Wilderness of Size.
>
> By Death's bold Exhibition
> Preciser what we are
> And the Eternal function
> Enabled to infer. (J856/Fr1092)

Where am I now on this latest journey through the labyrinth of grief? Past the "Hour of Lead," past the "formal feeling," past those days when I had to concentrate on the smallest chores to hold myself together.

> Therefore — we do life's labor —
> Though life's Reward — be done —
> With scrupulous exactness —
> To hold our Senses — on — (J443/Fr522)

Life is beginning to make sense—not entirely, but mostly, and in some changed way. Emily knew this experience too.

> We grow accustomed to the Dark —
> When Light is put away —
> As when the Neighbor holds the Lamp
> To witness her Good bye —
>
> A Moment — We uncertain step
> For newness of the night —
> Then — fit our Vision to the Dark —
> And meet the Road — erect —
>
> And so of larger — Darknesses —
> Those Evenings of the Brain —
> When not a Moon disclose a sign —
> Or Star — come out — within —
>
> The Bravest — grope a little —
> And sometimes hit a Tree
> Directly in the Forehead —
> But as they learn to see —
>
> Either the Darkness alters —
> Or something in the sight
> Adjusts itself to Midnight —
> And Life steps almost straight. (J419/Fr428)

Along with the sadness, along with feeling "almost straight," my life feels enriched in some very basic way, mellowed, ready for the new, aware that it will come.

Here I am.

Not knowing when the Dawn will come,
I open every Door, . . . (J1619/Fr1647)

NOTE

1. Joan Didion, *The Year of Magical Thinking* (New York: Knopf, 2005), 27–28.

Art has always been my salvation. My gods are Herman Melville, Mozart and Emily Dickinson. I believe in them with all my heart. I have a little, tiny Emily Dickinson book that I carry in my pocket everywhere. She is so strong. She is such a sexy, passionate woman. And when I am anxious, or worried about something, I read her words and I feel at peace.

MAURICE SENDAK, ILLUSTRATOR AND AUTHOR

September 2006

"An Element of Blank"
On Pain and Experimentation

CYNTHIA HOGUE

I know of no more accurate representations of pain than those found in Emily Dickinson. In "Pain—has an Element of Blank," for example, Dickinson writes of the self's infinitely narrowed horizons.

Pain — has an Element of Blank —
It cannot recollect
When it begun — or if there were
A time when it was not —

It has no Future — but itself
Its Infinite contain
It's Past — enlightened to perceive
New Periods — Of Pain. (J650/Fr760)

Any distinction we might want to draw between emotional and physical pain is rendered impossibly superfluous by that reifying pronoun, "it." Pain is a thing with a life of its own: it *is*. Pain posits us in an infinity of present tense that has no future but itself, containing both a past it cannot remember and us in a body of pain.

Of physical pain (of both torture and illness) Elaine Scarry has said that "physical suffering destroys language."[1] Suffering silences us. As Harold Schweizer asks in his study of suffering and art, "If suffering is in the unbearable, silent body rather than in the sharable, disembodied language of its narratives, how then can suffering speak? How can one hear the unspeakable? How can one listen without assuming one has understood? Indeed, how can one *begin* to

All citations of Dickinson's poems used in this chapter are from *The Poems of Emily Dickinson*, ed. R. W. Franklin, 3 vols. (Cambridge, Mass.: Harvard Univ. Press, 1998).

understand?"[2] The answer Schweizer suggests, that literature "might echo the mysterious occurrence of suffering,"[3] is itself anticipated by Dickinson's poem. Adrienne Rich, suffering from an excruciatingly painful and often disfiguring chronic illness, rheumatoid arthritis, agrees: "That is one property of poetic language: to engage with states that themselves would deprive us of language and reduce us to passive sufferers."[4]

Diagnosed some years ago with the same illness that Rich has, I had the uncanny experience of having studied her work closely without ever having concentrated on her representations of illness and pain. In fact, I did not even notice them. Rich's project in the 1980s and more recently has been persistently to learn "from the edges that blur" between "the body's pain and the pain on the streets," as she writes in her long poem "Contradictions: Tracking Poems."[5] Although she exhorts readers of that poem "who love clear edges" to "watch the edges that blur," I never heard her. I wrote much of my criticism on both Dickinson and Rich before becoming ill, and it was, as I say, uncanny to realize how, in their work, I routinely elided all references to a specific, localized pain, tracking instead the tormented, historically situated syntax of the body politic.

I was remarkably blind to *any* chronically ill body's specificity. Like others writing about Adrienne Rich, I mapped her search for a language honest and accurate enough to express her evolving feminist vision, which I argued produced formal innovations, what Elizabeth Meese calls dialogic "contra/dictions."[6] I sailed past images of "wrecked cartilage" and "elective surgery," consistently casting anchor at the broad picture's harbor: if a speaker "came out of the hospital," I focused on how she emerged "like a woman / who'd watched a massacre."[7] Thus, even as I sought passages emblematic of a divided, "contra/dictory" subject, I could not "see to see," to adapt Dickinson's well-known phrase that imaginatively tracks the process of dying (J465/Fr591). Critically, epistemologically, experientially, Rich's references to personal physical pain didn't exist for me.

But this blind spot is, as it turns out, the norm and not the exception. Bodies not in pain, that cannot physically feel the suffering, often stop at that imaginative chasm between them and the body in pain, unable to make the projective leap of empathy. For those bodies, suffering remains alien, opaque, closed to epistemological inquiry, to wit, clinically or *scientifically unconfirmed*. "Pain comes unsharably into our midst," Scarry writes, "as at once that which cannot be denied and that which cannot be confirmed."[8] For bodies in pain, Schweizer recounts, physical suffering is irreducible and unrepresentable, a dis/figuring inaccessibility to figuration: "Here at wit's end, at the point of a veritable epistemological crisis, is the moment of artistic, hermeneutical, or narrative beginning, the beginning of reading and writing."[9]

And so, reader, I began, although admittedly not with an empathetic, revelatory epiphany but from my own experience of chronic illness. For over two years, I reached "wit's end" in concrete if imperceptible ways to all but my closest friends and family. I lost the ability to write poetry and to read with any focus because of neurological symptoms not commonly associated with rheumatoid arthritis. It got extremely difficult to teach—I routinely forgot lesson plans or what I had intended to say or had already said (stopping dead mid-sentence). As the pain of my physical symptoms worsened, I also manifested personality changes from these clinically unconfirmed and medically undiagnosable symptoms. For the many doctors I consulted, my neuropathy simply did not exist.

My perspective was experiential, and therefore the symptoms did exist. The diminishment of cognitive skills was real—and for me, really problematic! I began to think I had Alzheimer's or perhaps early menopause. My short-term memory grew so bad that I forgot a poetry reading I was to give, brought the wrong student's master's thesis to a defense, drove across the Mississippi (when living in New Orleans) because I forgot to get off at my exit (in fact, could no longer remember why I had gotten into the car), became very dyslexic, and grew eerily obsessive. Whatever it was took "me," my identity as a writer and teacher, away. There was no one left, just some body. Dickinson's words helped me to share the unsharable, to speak the unspeakable in my poems.

BODY SCANS

Almost comforting, cradling &
claustrophobic, the metal
tube surrounds you
with driving sound, your head strapped
down so nothing moves. A voice
floats through the little mike:
"All right in there? Are you still
all right?" You're told half
an hour but it's fifty minutes.
Cold, you're hurtling
in space toward Mars,
chanting though you know
they hear you as they scan
your brain, deeper than the sea
& differing from God
as syllable from sound.

Later, when you huddle
on a metal table, they place
your feet, hands on a graph,
take pictures to see you
through & through.
Light cast from above
the machine marks
you with a cross,
a slanted star, a stained
glass window of a church.
"Don't breathe," they call,
                          & you don't.

As this poem suggests, I recall this time in my life with a still-symptomatic disassociation, a Dickinsonian "Element of Blank," and once the rheumatoid arthritis grew pronounced, an eternal present and presence of physical pain, "itself— / It's Infinite contain" (J650/Fr760). Words cannot comfort at a time like this, but the fact of their presence, their accompanying me through this time, was a line cast to the drowning.

In the following poem, as I tried (long after the worst pain had thankfully receded) to "contain" that sense of pain's infinity within the space of a sonnet, Dickinson's words again returned to me at a time when I was all but wordless. In some essential way, they were the gift her poetry gives, a gift that gives rather than takes.

THE NERVES LIKE TOMBS

As if an island under fog, memory's
outline blurs in fall and disappears
in spring. A broken chrysalis, the soul
dries up, self-emptied. When I
drive through town, I do not see
a stop light that I hurtle (deadly)
past to find myself crossing the river
out of town. I don't know why I stutter
or sentence stops and words like crows
wheel, cawing, away. One fears
for a self, but I have no fears
for this no-more being, this body-shell

with nothing-left to say. *First chill,*
then Stupor.   Then the letting go.

Susan Sontag writes that "illness is *not* a metaphor, and . . . the most truthful
way of regarding illness—and the healthiest way of being ill—is one most purified of, most resistant to, metaphoric thinking."[10] But how to approximate the
lived experience of illness in words that might convey how it feels? Rich's work,
arguably purified of metaphoric thinking about pain, has caused critics to ask
if such imagistically spare yet detailed accounts of the "medicalized body"[11]
should even be called poetry. But Lynda Bundtzen contends, "Rich knows the
risks she takes" when she offers "her body as a metaphorical vehicle for the
'body's world.'"[12] What's a writer to do when her body is, as Rich writes, "sig-
nified by pain"?[13] For one to face illness, it must not be transformed into something other than what it is, but the ill body takes us out of ourselves, points us
to larger ills than those of any individual.

Like Dickinson before her, Rich has approached the pain of others by bearing witness to her own.[14] Her testimonial poetry constitutes an action, as I
have argued elsewhere,[15] albeit a verbal one, or a "performative *speech act,*" as
Shoshana Felman characterizes such action.[16] The act of bearing witness (an at
times excruciatingly solitary responsibility) forces the witness to address *some-*
one, to seek out and sometimes to be possessed by a responsive "you."[17] The
final poem in Rich's *Dark Fields of the Republic,* "Edgelit," for example, inhabits
the point of view of the Northern Irish poet Medbh McGuckian, as well as her
voice, as it collages-in a portion of a letter McGuckian has written to Rich.

> *one's poetry seems aimless*
>
> *covered in the blood and lies*
>
> *oozing corrupt & artificial*
>
> *but of course one will continue . . .*

By positioning herself as addressee in the poem, Rich is able to posit herself not
only as listener-witness but as speaker-respondent, pronouncing into being poetry as an alternative to, and outside the concerns of, the death drive: "Medbh,
poetry means refusing / the choice to kill or die."[18] If chronic physical pain did
not allow Rich another site from which to speak, at least for a long time, she has
tried to solve that problem of the self's absorption into pain by being imaginatively "possessed" and haunted by others' pain.

Unlike Rich and Dickinson, I lost much of my cognitive capacity; like them,
I lost my physical well-being at the same time that I became despairingly aware

of the *greater* pain of others in the world, about which I could do nothing. The following poem tracks the form of that feeling:

AMONG PAIN

For the body possibly to have gone through,
of the minutest and crucial sensations,
each having its purpose, or configuration:
In the mind everything goes, larger than sky
or God, the heft of all being in perception,

the weight of weight, of sense the same
only through feelings everyone shares:
"I" does not seem unbelievable nor events improbable.
Pain bleeds through imagination, unimaginative:
it just is. One wishes to do something, go somewhere,

but everywhere the sensation remains,
the body in pain. Its eyes look
on fuchsia and lilac overtaking
the back fence, it still bleeds,
and *I* am knowing this

(body that cannot rise
from its chair,
that never weeps,
in earth's house-
hold of pain).

My mind scrolls through a list of disappeared,
decimated beings. If there is no escape,
no separation, there are also no lies.
Sun shines on the arid soil of this garden.
Pain blooms in a body. Blossoms without water.

As all the orienting markers by which I knew myself dissolved, moreover, and I no longer had any sense of myself except through a few labels (which had once seemed so internalized but were revealed to me as external labels only—"teacher," "writer"), I found myself changed and humbled. As I had to let go of all hopes of normative action, I also had to release that old and vanished self. The process became for me, in the way of other traumatizing experiences, transformative. Call it a spiritual or ethical journey—or perhaps Julia Kristeva's notion of "herethics" is most apt, since in order to write at all, I had to find new ways of writing (for there was no longer a "self" to express). Of the "herethical" function of art, Kristeva writes, "[artistic] practice is ethical when it dissolves those narcissistic fixations (ones that are narrowly confined to the subject) to which the signifying process succumbs in its socio-symbolic realization." For Kristeva, this "practice" of "dissolving . . . the unity of the subject" is ethical because it resists an other-denying self-absorption that some would argue is exemplified by the unified and monologic subject that dominates lyric tradition.[19]

As a poet without words, I was finally able to begin to write again by allowing the words of others to come to my aid. I employed the methods of quotation and collage that Rich and another poet whose work I'd studied critically, Marianne Moore, had used to formally radical effects. Moore, I had once argued, creatively recontextualizes the "found language" she quotes (often without attribution, and usually from noncanonical sources).[20] A poetic bricolage of sorts, as Margaret Holley aptly describes Moore's methodology, her "hybrid method" produces not a different sort of poem, but a hybrid — a cross between two generic boundaries.[21] Her method of collage and assemblage liberated me to write at a time when I had no one to express. Without my ventriloquizing Dickinson, the poet who "[lit] but Lamps" as if for me alone (J883/Fr930), I would not have found my way along that difficult path or discovered out of my own incapacitation a capacity for being, a larger listening among words.

NOTES

An earlier version of this essay is included in "Titanic Operas" on the Emily Dickinson Electronic Archives Web site, curated by Martha Nell Smith (http://www.emilydickinson.org/main_toc.html). Some of this essay was included as part of a longer personal essay titled "The Tao of Disease," *Poetry International* 4 (2000): 123–33. Excerpts from the title sequence, "The Incognito Body," are now collected in *The Incognito Body* (Los Angeles: Red Hen Press, 2006)and are quoted with permission of the author. I wish to thank Cindy MacKenzie for her editorial vision. I would also like to thank Martha Nell Smith of the Dickinson Electronic Archives and Federico Moramarco of *Poetry International* for their encouragement and support.

1. Elaine Scarry, *The Body in Pain: The Making and Unmaking of the World* (New York: Oxford Univ. Press, 1985), 201.

2. Harold Schweizer, *Suffering and the Remedy of Art* (Albany: State Univ. of New York Press, 1997), 12–13.

3. Ibid., 13.

4. Adrienne Rich, *What Is Found There* (New York: W. W. Norton, 1993), 10. For a discussion of this aspect of the poem, see Lynda K. Bundtzen, "Adrienne Rich's Identity Poetics: A Partly Common Language," *Women's Studies* 27.4 (1998): 331–45.

5. Adrienne Rich, *Your Native Land, Your Life: Poems* (New York and London: W. W. Norton, 1986), 88–111.

6. "Contra/dictions," according to Elizabeth A. Meese, denote the oppositions Rich puts into play and undoes in her attempts to work through the perceptions Jewish assimilation has affected. For Rich, Meese suggests, "the separation from the other is a separation within the self, requiring us to undertake multiple, unending negotiations with the logic of identity." See Elizabeth A. Meese, *(Ex)tensions: Re-Figuring Feminist Criticism* (Urbana and Chicago: Univ. of Illinois Press, 1990), 172, 173.

7. Rich, *Your Native Land*, 93, 111.

8. Scarry, 4.

9. Schweizer, 16.

10. Susan Sontag, *Illness as Metaphor and AIDS and Its Metaphors* (New York: Picador / Farrar, Straus and Giroux, 2001), 3.

11. See Mary K. Deshazer, "Fractured Borders: Women's Cancer and Feminist Theatre," *NWSA Journal* 15.2 (Summer 2003): 5–26.

12. Bundtzen, 339.

13. Rich, *Your Native Land*, 89.

14. A voluntary or involuntary (or conscious or unconscious) "*appointment* to bear witness" is how Felman and Laub describe the subject position of the contemporary, testimonial writer. See Shoshana Felman and Dori Laub, *Testimony: Crises of Witnessing in Literature, Psychoanalysis, and History* (New York: Routledge, 1992), 3 (emphasis in the original).

15. See Cynthia Hogue, "Adrienne Rich's Political, Ecstatic Subject," *Women's Studies* 27.4 (1998): 413–29.

16. Of the dynamic of testimony, Felman and Laub assert that to "*produce* one's own speech as material evidence for truth . . . is to accomplish a *speech act,* rather than to simply formulate a [poetic] statement": "As a performative speech act, testimony in effect addresses what in history is *action* that exceeds any substantialized significance, and what in happenings is *impact* that dynamically explodes any conceptual reifications and any constative delimitations." See Felman and Laub, *Testimony,* 5.

17. Felman and Laub write that "by virtue of the fact that the testimony is *addressed* to others, the witness, from within the solitude of [her] own stance, is the vehicle of an occurrence, a reality, a stance or dimension *beyond [herself].*" See Felman and Laub, *Testimony,* 3 (emphasis in the original).

18. Adrienne Rich, *Dark Fields of the Republic: Poems 1991–1995* (New York: W. W. Norton, 1995), 70, 71 (Rich's lineation, italics, and ellipsis). I take this opportunity to thank my former colleague, Joyce scholar John Rickard from Bucknell University, whom I consulted on Irish women's poetry when writing this section, for whose expertise on Irish poetry in general and Irish women's poetry in particular I was most grateful.

19. Julia Kristeva, *Revolution in Poetic Language*, trans. Margaret Waller (New York: Columbia Univ. Press, 1987), 232–33.

20. See Cynthia Hogue, *Scheming Women: Poetry, Privilege, and the Politics of Subjectivity* (Albany: State Univ. of New York Press, 1995), 73–116.

21. Margaret Holley, *The Poetry of Marianne Moore: A Study in Voice and Value* (New York: Cambridge Univ. Press, 1987), 38.

Elements of Blank, Formal Feelings, and an Autobiography of Chronic Pain

MARTHA NELL SMITH

PROLOGUE

Discussions about pain in Emily Dickinson's poetry almost always focus on psychic, emotional experience, as if her literary attentions to physical pain are emblems or metaphors for estates of the heart, spirit, or mind. Just as often, the topic of pain or suffering in her works is conflated with that of death. Emotional anguish is frequently assumed to be what she means to conjure by painful physical images, scenes, and expressions: emotional distress is assumed to be the cause of such poetic articulations. In other words, vocabularies of pain are, as it is often presumed about the pain itself, symptoms of something really wrong in realms other than the physical. I do not doubt that Emily Dickinson writes about emotional, spiritual, sexual, erotic, and mental anguishes, nor do I question that she uses physical metaphors to depict those. But those particular slants of attention are not the subject of this autobiographical sketch of chronic pain.

Sometimes physical pain is all and only itself, so engulfing an agony that it consumes emotional, spiritual, sexual, mental, *all* response that it begets. Sometimes physical pain, chronic pain, is *that* overwhelming, and that realm of suffering is awful—awe-full—and a very lonely place to be. For decades now I have walked with Emily Dickinson. My first volume of her words is tattered and falls to pieces when I take it down from the shelf. That she took the practically unfathomable, unameliorable, unrelievable realm of physical hurt as a poetic subject has been tender comfort in many a dark sweat of nights agonistes. From those caverns of throbbing pain, my beloved partner, and also our fabulous dog, seemed so comfortable, resting in slumber as my arthritic limb cracked, cracking me. Harvard English professor Elaine Scarry, a literary theorist and cultural

All citations of Dickinson's poems used in this chapter are from *The Manuscript Books of Emily Dickinson,* ed. R. W. Franklin (Cambridge, Mass.: Harvard Univ. Press, 1981).

critic widely regarded for her acute analyses of pain and, especially in the wake of September 11, 2001, her examination of terrorism, observes that "as physical pain destroys the mental content and language of the person in pain, so it also tends to appropriate and destroy the conceptualization abilities and language of persons who only observe the pain."[1] She echoes Dickinson's "There is a pain — so utter — / It swallows substance up" (J599/Fr 515), and in reading an academic treatise I find myself swimming in the memory of poetry comforting enough and strong enough to trust to. *Utter:* situated on the outside or extreme limit; remote and often most remote from the center; carried to the utmost point or highest degree; extreme to the point of strangeness or abnormality. Strangeness? Abnormality? Yes, at first this is the case with pain that overtakes one. But as Dickinson knew, pain so utter and excruciating becomes being, becomes, though it seems perverse to write it, udder or suckle to one's being. That Dickinson braves this subject at all is on the one hand astonishing. Yet this poet whose ambitions aimed to plumb human experience had no choice but to write of this state of consciousness, of "physical pain" that—"unlike any other state of consciousness—has no referential content. It is not *of* or *for* anything. It is precisely because it takes no object that it, more than any other phenomenon, resists objectification in language."[2] The exploration of this essay, then, is of the subject of physical pain, chronic physical pain, my prison of pain, and the friend I found during that period in Emily Dickinson.

THE BODY

On December 13, 1994, after three and a half hours of surgery, my orthopedic surgeon declared the hip replacement a success, having lengthened my left leg 3.5 centimeters, to within three to four millimeters the length of my right leg. He had drilled into what remained of the hip bone, the arthritically diseased portions of which he had cut away, and successfully secured the new custom-designed titanium, cobalt, and plastic joint and socket. He told his team to prepare to close and removed the clamps from the leg's major vein and artery. Shocked, the young orthopedic resident, Penny Stringer, watched in horror as the English professor whose history she had taken early that morning crashed, suddenly without blood pressure. Five units of blood rushed out immediately. The teams struggled for hours to pump up my pressure, stabilize me, keep my life from draining away with my corpuscles. My vein was in tatters, severed raggedly, and my artery nicked, thus my bleeding out was both a gush and a trickle. As it has been since late afternoon of that fateful 13th, now my vein is tied off and a graft facilitates the artery's flow of blood. To prevent scar tissue from clogging up my blood flow, a baby aspirin every day is my prescription, far different from the narcotic Percocet, which I, a body always in pain, lived on for almost all of 1994.

. . .

It was not Emily Dickinson poems that she sang to me when I awoke in intensive care eight hours after my awful crash on the operating table, the ventilator still in. Leaning over me, murmuring what the nurses had been saying—"You had a very hard time in surgery, but you're going to be OK. You're stable now. They'll take the breathing device out soon"—my partner didn't sing Emily Dickinson poems but a Bruce Springsteen anthem: "Oh-oh come take my hand / we're riding out tonight to case the promised land / oh-oh Thunder Road, oh Thunder Road / oh Thunder Road. . . . Show a little faith, there's magic in the night. . . ." Just as she had ten months earlier, walking me down the mountain after my nasty wrist-breaking fall, carrying my cross-country skis, she sang the entire song—". . . Hey what else can we do now? / Except roll down the window / and let the wind blow / back your hair / Well the night's bustin' open / These two lanes will take us anywhere. . . ." This time she sang softly into my ear as I stared at the clock on the wall, knowing something awful had happened. Otherwise I wouldn't be in intensive care. I was not breathing on my own and was frustrated not to be able to talk over the ventilator, but I wasn't ready for them to take it out yet. All I felt that night was the machine forcing air into my lungs and thirst, awful thirst that somehow felt cold, and cool trickles down my throat as the crushed ice melted. All I knew was that something was missing.

When all sixteen doctors who were in that operating room came to see me the next day—the orthopedic team, the anesthesia team, the vascular team, the neurology team—orthopedic resident Penny Stringer, who knew the English professor had written two books on Emily Dickinson, lingered for just a moment after her team departed and gave me the calligraphy copy of "I dwell in Possibility" that she had stayed up all night making. "We're not supposed to do this, but you're so young, and we were all so shaken." "The spreading wide my narrow Hands / To gather Paradise" (J657/Fr466) was all I could quote of the poem at that weak but relieved moment. Dr. Stringer smiled, "I'm glad you're here." And I knew, even at that hazy moment, that a possibility I believed unobtainable had indeed been realized. Through all the anesthesia, through all the terror of awakening in ICU and knowing I was attached to a machine to help me breath, I knew what was missing—the deep pain that had become so integral to my identity. That deep, gnawing, relentless pain was missing, gone.

. . .

In May 1990, having given a talk about Susan and Emily Dickinson's lifelong passion for one another and for poetry—"sermon — hope — solace — life"[3]—at Columbia University and walking on New York's Upper West Side the next day with dear friends, I stepped off a curb and felt a searing, wrenching, previously unimaginable pain. Ironically unimaginable because it was a pain I had known but which I had forgotten. A pain so harrowing, so debilitating, that it can only be "remembered" when one is in its maelstrom. Outside that maelstrom, memory, sweet friend, "covers the Abyss with Trance" (J599/Fr515). Yet that Manhattan afternoon, pain exploded out of the low-grade, amazing bruised constancy, my nine-year trance that enabled " . . . Memory [to] step / Around — across — upon it." That inner explosion, inaudible to the dear friends and dearest companion walking with me, was transport, and pain brought me face-to-face with memory and back to a soft summer night in 1981 and a wreck off the highway, "As one within a Swoon — / Goes safely — where an Open Eye — / Would drop Him — Bone by Bone" (J599/Fr515).

Pain "remembered" before; pain on the order of the crack that threw my consciousness's eye open as it ripped across my femur when I awoke, bloody and desperate, and tried to get out of the crumpled car. Pain on the order of the crack that threw my consciousness's eye open as it ripped across my femur while I stood before my class at Rutgers University in January 1983. There, my imperfectly "healed" bone broke apart, gouging nerves . . . again. I stared fiercely and my students stared right back, afraid to do anything but what I asked them to do—leave, and go get help. Immediately. Pain that "cannot recollect / When it begun—Or if there were / A time when it was not" (J650/Fr760/MB34, p. 819). I had first become acquainted with that excruciation on June 21, 1981, as I lay in a car at the bottom of a New Jersey ravine, dying. I was a young woman in her twenties, driving alone on a winding New Jersey mountain road, returning from a party thrown in my honor, proud of my moderation as far as libations were concerned. Too arrogant, foolhardy, and immoderate to wear a seatbelt, I was absolutely confident when my right front wheel went off the tarmac and I turned the steering wheel sharply to get all four tires firmly back on the road. I was on a steep sharp curve and in my blithe assurance did not notice—until it was much too late—that my correction was overwrought. In a split second I was crashing through and out the thick country-roadside brush. Momentarily airborne, I could fly! But the landing two hundred feet down was nasty, much too hard, too crushing for me to remember. I do recall waking up, choking on my own blood, spotting the lights of a party from the mansion tucked on the other side of this affluent hill. I will go to them, get help, I thought. All will be

OK. When I tried to leave the car, pain seared, soared, immobilized, and I knew that there is indeed no pain quite like that of a broken bone. "It has no Future — but itself — / It's Infinite contain / It's Past — Enlightened to / perceive / New Periods — Of Pain" (J650/Fr760). An "Element of Blank," an endorphin-pumped mindfulness so acute, so intent on relieving the consciousness, that it euphorically bears an especial mindlessness toward the pain. An Element of Blank that cannot know because it can only know, Pain. A pain that can remark the day of the concussive irrevocable and so "knows" its beginning but has no real memory of life without pain.

> After great pain, a formal feeling comes.
> If that is the case, then after great happiness
> Should a feeling come that is somehow informal?[4]

Emily Dickinson inspires such complex humor, as Alicia Ostriker's "Poem Beginning with a Line by Dickinson" illustrates. The poet responding to Dickinson injects emotion into being in and out of pain, but, as in Dickinson's poem, there is no referent for pain and none for happiness either. "The Nerves sit ceremonious, like Tombs" (J341/Fr372), but why? What does it mean that the feeling, having just "come," seems then to take on a life, a volition of its own? So separate has this pain become that it requires the third-person pronoun, a dissociation from the first-person singular. Supple, athletic "Feet" are "mechanical" and go nowhere but "round" on terra less and less firm, from "Air" to "Ought." Wood becomes fossilized, "Quartz," "stone." Time is counted in the "Hour of Lead"—in terms of the dull, cold metal; a plummet for sounding; a thin strip of metal used to separate lines of type in print; the turn of a screw? "Remembered, if outlived" only in the "letting go" of everything one outside of the pain thinks it might be "*of* or *for.*" In this, Dickinson attempts to create a material record, an artifact that casts pain, sentient experience, out of the "privacy of the human interior"[5] and into the visible world.

That she thought long and hard about the importance of "letting go" in pain is obvious in the manuscript version of the following poem.

> The hallowing of Pain
> Like hallowing of Heaven,
> Obtains at a Corporeal
> Cost —
> The Summit is not given

To Him who strives
severe
At + Middle of the Hill —
But He who has
Achieved the + Top —
All — is the price
of All —

+ Bottom—Centre + Crest — (J772/Fr 871/MB39, p. 952)

With the simple change of an alphabetic letter, a slightly different stroke of the pen, "Hallowing" becomes "Harrowing," an orthographic proximity surely not lost on Dickinson. And in this the old adages—pain builds character, makes one a stronger person—are revealed as the overly simple, if well-intended, empty exhortations that they are. Such adages can only be uttered from outside pain, from outside knowing, for as Dickinson's variant choices make starkly clear— "Middle," "Bottom," "Centre," "Top," "Crest"—the senses of direction that order experience are not distinctly decipherable in this world of pain where "All — is the price / of All" and where price and purchase thus become meaningless. In this, the Christian assertion that suffering on earth is the "price" to purchase eternal bliss in "Heaven" is laid bare in all its insensitivity—pain is itself and only itself, outside all systems of knowing and reckoning, even our arbitrary measures for time. "Pain — expands the Time — / Ages coil within / The minute circumference / Of a single Brain — // Pain contracts — the Time — / Occupied with Shot / Gamuts of Eternities / Are as they were not" (J967/Fr833).

CODA

Is happiness, then, the body out of pain? To say that the subject of this paper is physical pain and not emotional, spiritual, mental, erotic pain is of course an impossible dream, as Emily Dickinson's poems about pain, as well as long-standing interpretations of them that assert the emotional, spiritual, mental, and erotic, make clear. The world of pain seems to those outside it, even to those who have once been in it, a world of dream, or nightmare. Those in pain pray for release from the dream/nightmare because that netherworld is consciousness apart or within, not consciousness subsumed, overtaken, all in all.

I am not a fantastic dreamer and often joke that it amazes me that I can stay asleep during my own dreams, which tend to be far from profound, occupied as they are with selecting just the right tomato sauce from the shelf of a Whole Foods grocery or with some other mundane task. But a couple of weeks after I came home from the hospital in late 1994, just in time for the holidays, I had a dream about a conference very much like those held for literary congregants such as the annual meetings of the Emily Dickinson International Society. In this dream I was catching the bus, perhaps to dash from one conference hotel to another or to go to the airport. I'm not really sure and it doesn't really matter. With my suit bag hanging on my shoulder, I stood in the pouring rain, waiting for the bus. As I leapt onto the bus, my suit bag was suddenly swept away in the torrent, swept down, down, and away into the rushing waters of the storm drain. I leapt off the crowded bus, screaming after the suit bag, knowing and awakening in that knowledge that it was gone forever. I awoke in that resignation, knowing I had lost something. Something was missing. I was, for the first time in thirteen years, a body free from chronic pain.

I still do not know how to talk about that "Element of Blank." And so I am reminded of just how desperately we need the poets, and why I have walked all these years with Emily Dickinson.

NOTES

1. Elaine Scarry, *The Body in Pain: The Making and Unmaking of the World* (New York: Oxford Univ. Press, 1985), 279.

2. Ibid., 5.

3. In an undated letter to Curtis Hidden Page, Susan Huntington Dickinson makes the remarks quoted. The original documents can be found in the Papers of Susan Dickinson, Martha Dickinson Bianchi Collection, Brown University Libraries. The letter is published online in *Writings by Susan Dickinson,* ed. Martha Nell Smith, Laura Lauth, and Lara Vetter, at http://www.emilydickinson. org/susan/chp1.html. Available 1999 to present.

4. Alicia Ostriker, *The Imaginary Lover* (Pittsburgh: Univ. of Pittsburgh Press, 1986), 57.

5. Scarry, 280.

Life Portals

LINDA RICHARD

In the first years after my son died in 1998, I couldn't go near the section of a bookstore or library that might contain a book or books about the loss of a child. And although I am a "book person" with thousands of cherished volumes in my personal library, no one in my life thought to give me such a book. But messages came from one friend via e-mail that provided a connection to the pain of others that made me feel less alone. This friend, Cindy, was a classmate I met in graduate school in Suzanne Juhasz's seminar on Emily Dickinson at the University of Colorado in the early nineties. Years later, after Brandon's death, Cindy periodically sent me lines of Dickinson poetry, lines without explanation or explication, her message without greeting or lament. I printed the e-mails and tacked them to my bulletin board. They are lines that most lovers of Dickinson's poetry know by heart. It was a relief to receive these familiar lines. Here were words that addressed the magnitude of my loss. I couldn't go to Dickinson myself yet. She had to come to me, via my friend.

> I like a look of Agony,
> Because I know it's true.... (J241/Fr339)

> I can wade Grief —
> Whole Pools of it —
> I'm used to that —
> But the least push of Joy.... (J252/Fr312)

> 'Tis the Seal Despair —

All citations of Dickinson's poems used in this chapter are from *The Poems of Emily Dickinson,* ed. Thomas H. Johnson, 3 vols. (Cambridge, Mass.: Harvard Univ. Press, 1955).

An imperial affliction
Sent us of the Air. . . . (J258/Fr320)

This is the Hour of Lead —
Remembered, if outlived,
As Freezing persons, recollect the Snow —
First — Chill — then Stupor — then the letting go — (J341/Fr372)

Cindy didn't try to make it better, though sometimes she did remind me to "try to 'dwell in Possibility'" (J657/Fr466), to remain open to a lessening of anguish during my "awful leisure" (J1100/Fr1100). Despite the darkness I descended into after Brandon's sudden death, Cindy coaxed me to observe, if only momentarily, a vibrancy from the past, a love of Emily Dickinson's work she knew we both shared. It was a slender thread. A lifeline. In graduate school, Cindy and I often had long conversations about how the poet of another time and place was with us the way a living friend would be—she sat at our lunch table and walked with us along campus footpaths. I wrote a poem about a solitary, unexpected meeting with Dickinson.

WAKING EARLY TO EMILY DICKINSON ON HER BIRTHDAY
We talked with each other about each other
Though neither of us spoke. . . .
Emily Dickinson (J1473/Fr1506)

Not winter in
December, not yet.

Strands of fog emerge
in tangles, waking
from a night beneath cypress
rising to skies not leaden
but jasper and silver—raw
silk falls back from fingers
long, that trace the fine

Intrusion of your face
where the mountain breaks
or where fog fills up
the seam of air I breathe.

From more than a hundred
years away, time serving
our purpose now

A wisp of veil
lifts to allow
this meeting
an economy of cosmic
celebration—not
longing for you
but living you

In the morning
in December.

There are those who write that Emily Dickinson's poetry is about survival, that through the process of turning sorrow into art she transcends her circumstance. We seem to write about survival as if it were in itself a raison d'être. Parents whose children have died don't believe they should live on. Recently I listened to the grown-up daughter of a dying friend say that she knew as a child that she had to be very careful because if anything had ever happened to her, her father would not have survived. So, by her diligence, she secured her father's life.

I wanted to ask her, So what happens when a child does die? What does a mother do if she loves her child as much as I loved mine? She needs to die, of course. There is no hope of survival here. Living is an affront to love, to the will that rises up in every caring parent to protect her child, to keep him safe. If a parent fails? There is no redemption for this failure.

Psychologist Judith Bernstein, in her book *When the Bough Breaks: Forever after the Death of a Son or Daughter*, writes, "An orphan is a child without a parent. A widow or widower is a person who has lost a spouse. . . . There is no word to identify to the outside world a parent who has lost a child. Perhaps the concept is too unthinkable."[1]

In these nine years since my son's death, I have experienced a cascade of other losses. Another child, Coco, who came to me as an eighteen-year-old babysitter for my three children one summer and stayed as part of my family (her own mom had died of cancer when Coco was twelve years old)—this beloved daughter died of breast cancer last year. She was thirty-seven. And I have lost three friends from my life's inner circle within the past two years, all of them dying of cancer, and all of them too young to leave, it seems to me. What I did not foresee as I bore witness to their suffering and struggled with my own was a tender evolution in me: the miraculous can rise up out of sorrow to infuse everything that grows, every life, every breath with a shimmering—a way of seeing with compassion and deeper insight that takes nothing for granted. I know I can't really "be alive" with the innocence I once felt, but I have entered into a new kind of being through the life portal that Emily Dickinson has given us, where I find meaning nonetheless. Dickinson writes, "Unto a broken heart / No other one may go / Without the high prerogative / Itself hath suffered too" (J1704/Fr1745). I can offer myself up as witness. This is what I hope my poem about Brandon conveys. The wild flowers are, of course, the very ones the poet would have gathered.

IN APRIL, NINE DAYS AFTER HIS 21ST BIRTHDAY . . .
Till ranks of seeds their witness bear —
And softly thro' the altered air
Emily Dickinson (J130/Fr122)

We dwell in a house of grief
Mother without a son
Young wife without a husband
Little girl without her daddy
Brother and sister with no brother between
Wailing walls faces press against

If onlies
and
Arms aching to
Hold him one more time
The grass is mowed, the sun
The sun
Shines down

The red dragonfly that hovered
Over the pool last summer returns
The wildflowers Brandon scattered as seeds
The June he married begin to bloom again in

Preposterous
Profusion—White Yarrow   Red

California Poppy   Black-eyed Susan
        Bluebell   Sweet William   Ox-eye Daisy   Blue
Flag Iris   Red Clover   White Sweet
        Clover   Cowslip   Spurred Snap Dragon   Red
Flax   Dame's Rocket   Yellow Lady's Slipper
        Lupine   Trillium   Cosmos   and
        Forget-me-not

Some waist high—
Brandon being Brandon
Barefoot
Running through them

Notes

1. Judith R. Bernstein, *When the Bough Breaks: Forever after the Death of a Son or Daughter* (Kansas City, Mo.: Andrews McMeel, 1997), 168.

Imaginative literature is otherness, and as such alleviates loneliness.

HAROLD BLOOM

I bear witness to Dickinson's intellectual and spiritual ascendancy. Her poetry taught itself to eight of my recent classes, graduate and under-graduate alike. Although my publications to date have elicited only the mildest curiosity from nonacademics—an alumni magazine article or two, the odd feature in local news outlets—I have encountered Dickinson fans in supermarkets. At a family reunion, the other attendee who fielded questions about his or her work, albeit as a sideshow to the main event of football, was my cousin the doctor. If only I could prove equal to satisfy-ing sharp curiosity about Dickinson. When all else fails, I say that reading Dickinson's poems is like eating peanuts, or more formally, "Ho, everyone that thirsteth, come ye to the waters, and he that hath no money; come ye, buy, and eat; yea, come; buy wine and milk without money and without price" (Isaiah 55:1).

RICHARD BRANTLEY
Experience and Faith: The Late-Romantic Imagination of Emily Dickinson
(New York: Palgrave/Macmillan Press, 2004)

"A crescent still abides"

Emily Dickinson and the Work of Mourning

Joan Kirkby

There are days when I can't read Emily Dickinson. I can't go near her—which is a strange thing to say in a book about the healing power of Dickinson's poetry, but it's true. Poems like "The first Day's Night had come" (J410/Fr423) or "The Soul has Bandaged moments" (J512/Fr360) or "I tried to think a lonelier Thing" (J532/Fr570) or "To fill a Gap" (J546/Fr647) are strictly off limits. And yet, even in the darkest times, those times when I don't want to read her, I know she's there, a constant companion and friend. And I know from her own testament that she has gone through this experience, that she has articulated it, that she has found reparation, and that, for her, it has become a source of wonder and of speculative thought. And what is this to-be-avoided "thing" that provokes my occasional fear of Emily Dickinson? It is, quite simply, the spectre of death and irredeemable loss.

Grief seems to be one of the most disconcerting experiences we can have. It is certainly one of the most difficult to negotiate, to speak about and share, yet mourning that is unacknowledged or foreclosed can have devastating consequences. I think it is because, as Judith Butler has written, death and mourning are not optional; in grief, we do not stay "intact" but are given over to a "transformation . . . the full result of which one cannot know in advance."[1] Nevertheless, we are often told somewhat glibly by others—sometimes even close friends—to get over it or pull ourselves together. I can remember nearly twenty years ago telling a younger friend on the occasion of a particularly painful loss that I had now lost everyone without whom I thought I could not live. I also remember his recoiling from my words while at the same time thanking me for telling him, but in a highly ironic tone. I realized then that I had crossed

All citations of Dickinson's poems used in this chapter are from *The Poems of Emily Dickinson*, ed. R. W. Franklin, 3 vols. (Cambridge, Mass.: Harvard Univ. Press, 1998).

some unspoken boundary where it is almost never all right to speak of the inner world, and I thought of Dickinson's words.

> It's Hour with itself
> The Spirit never shows—
> What Terror would enthrall the Street
> Could Countenance disclose
>
> The Subterranean Freight
> The Cellars of the Soul —
> Thank God the loudest Place he made
> Is licensed to be still. (J1225/Fr1211)

Of course, my remark was naive and shortsighted, for there were more deaths
to come. There is always more death, and, in fact, the one thing that we have
to become skilled at is loss and "the work" of mourning. For each time we lose
someone we love, our world is utterly destroyed and we ourselves are subjected
to violent reconfiguration. With or without our consent, we are inevitably and
irrevocably transformed. And each time, a part of ourselves goes missing, as
Dickinson so beautifully describes on the occasion of the death of her friend
Otis Lord in March 1884.

> Each that we lose takes part of us;
> A crescent still abides,
> Which like the moon, some turbid night,
> Is summoned by the tides. (J1605/Fr1634)

Reading through Dickinson's poems and letters, it is clear that she consid-
ers dying to be a central and ongoing task: "'Tis Dying — I am doing — but /
I'm not afraid to know" (J692/Fr715). Who can ever forget their first reading of
Dickinson, her exuberance in the face of death and those provocative "drop-
dead" first lines: "If I shouldn't be alive / When the Robins come" (J182/Fr210);
"I felt a Funeral, in my Brain" (J280/Fr340); "'Twas just this time, last year, I
died" (J445/Fr344); "I died for Beauty — but was scarce / Adjusted in the Tomb"
(J449/Fr448); "I heard a Fly buzz — when I died" (J465/Fr591); "Because I could
not stop for Death — / He kindly stopped for me " (J712/Fr479). In speaking
so irreverently about death in the voice of those who have already experienced
that "Extension" (L650), the speakers in Dickinson's poetry find excitement and

a release of energy: "'Tis so appalling — it exhilarates" (J281/Fr341). For Dickinson, crisis is enlivening.

> A Bomb upon the Ceiling
> Is an improving thing —
> It keeps the nerves progressive
> Conjecture flourishing. . . . (J1128/Fr1150)

Similarly, she suggests that "The Dying" is a "Height" that "Reorganizes Estimate" and "'Tis Compound Vision — / Light — enabling Light — / The Finite — furnished / With the Infinite" (J906/Fr830).

It is not death in the abstract that Dickinson explores. It is the particular loss, which renders life numinous at the very moment that the self is impoverished. We know from psychoanalysis—from Freud and Klein and Abraham and Torok—that the death of a beloved person is a dangerous time for those left behind. Mourners often experiences an overwhelming desire to go with the one who has died, particularly if the death has been violent or unexpected, for then there is often a sense of urgency, a feeling that if they hurry, if their own death could be accelerated, they might still catch up with their loved one on the other side. They feel that they have lost an integral part of themselves, that a crucial piece of their internal puzzle is gone and they are left inconsolable, ravished, inchoate.

In classic accounts of mourning and melancholia, there is the evocation of an "open wound" that draws into itself all the negative energies of the world and empties the ego until it is totally impoverished.[2] This can give rise, in turn, to feelings of hatred and persecution in the bereaved.[3] In Abraham and Torok's account, there is an attempt to "hide, wall in, and encrypt" the wound from the rest of the psyche in "a crypt built with the bricks of hate and aggression."[4] There is also, inevitably, an element of disfiguration, as Judith Butler has suggested more recently: "I am wounded, and I find that the wound itself testifies to the fact that I am . . . given over to the Other in ways that I cannot fully predict or control"[5]—"It is not as if an 'I' exists independently over here and then simply loses a 'you' over there, especially if the attachment to 'you' is part of what composes who 'I' am."[6]

In his essay "Mourning and Melancholia" (1917), Freud emphasizes that mourning is work, perhaps the hardest work we ever undertake, and that mourning takes considerable time. The mental work that consumes the mourner is to revive, relive, and then to release and excise the myriad ties that connect us to the one we have lost. In profound mourning, there is a "loss of interest in the outside world—in so far as it does not recall him [who is lost]," a "loss of capacity to adopt any new object of love (which would mean replacing him)," and a "turning away from any activity that is not connected with thoughts of him."[7] In Freud's account "each single one of the memories and expectations" that attached us to the dead must be worked through—"bit by bit, at great expense of time and cathectic energy."[8] Ever so gradually—and the work of mourning is slow and painful and energy consuming—we must relinquish our attachment to the beloved and sever the poignant memories and images that tie us to them. But there is worse to come in this psychoanalytic account—there is a second death and a third—the beloved object must be relinquished and abandoned in order for the living to reconnect to the world of the living.

However, there are darker implications in the psychoanalytic account. The imperative to relinquish, abandon, and replace the dead is, in my view, experienced by the mourner as a kind of second death, and worse still this second death is one that must be "murderously" perpetrated by ourselves. It is as if the dead must be put to death by our own hand if we are to survive. And I think that it is the guilt born of this strenuous, impossible demand—that we must abandon the other if we are to go on living—that poses the most unbearable challenge to those in mourning. Nevertheless, this is the model that our culture has for the most part adopted. Not only have our loved ones died, if that were not enough, we must abandon them, and eventually we must forget them. As Dickinson writes, "There are those in the morgue that bewitch us with sweetness, but that which is dead must go with the ground" (L357). It is an intolerable predicament. After years of thinking through these classic essays on mourning and the experience of mourning itself, I think that it is the abhorrence of abandoning the now defenseless other and the guilt one feels as agent of this abandonment that are the most insufferable to the mourner. It is a terrible double bind; there is a battle within the psyche: who will live, who will die? Will the good self who is trying to keep the dead alive win, or the bad self who abandons the beloved to seek new attachments in the world of the living? What choice can we possibly make? It is no wonder, as Dickinson wrote, that "*Bareheaded life*—under the grass—worries one like a Wasp" (L220) or that so many of the interred speakers in Dickinson's poems still speak to us from beyond the grave.

Dickinson's sense of this murderous choice that lies at the heart of our being—to stay with the dead or to abandon them—gives her poetry its characteristic edginess. In "The last Night that She lived," the speaker conveys a sense of guilt in the presence of the dying, a guilt that she will be alive tomorrow while the one who is dying must "finish quite."

The last Night that She lived
It was a Common Night
Except the Dying—this to Us
Made Nature different

We noticed smallest things —
Things overlooked before
By this great light opon our Minds
Italicized — as 'twere.

As We went out and in
Between Her final Room
And Rooms where Those to be alive
Tomorrow were, a Blame

That others could exist
While She must finish quite
A Jealousy for Her arose
So nearly infinite —

We waited while She passed —
It was a narrow time —
Too jostled were Our Souls to speak
At length the notice came.

She mentioned, and forgot —
Then lightly as a Reed
Bent to the Water, struggled scarce —
Consented, and was dead —

And We — We placed the Hair —
And drew the Head erect —
And then an awful leisure was
Belief to regulate — (J1100/Fr1100)

The speaker is acutely aware of the brutal separation between the one who is dying and those who will be alive tomorrow. There is "a Blame // That Others could exist / While She must finish quite" that is not mitigated by the assertion of a "Jealousy for Her . . . So nearly infinite."

Dickinson's gothic poems enact what we might belatedly call the Freudian scene, though her work on mourning anticipates that of Freud by over fifty years. Death, madness, dissolution, and unbearable loss, "the Thief ingredient" (L359), she called it: "Looking at Death, is Dying" (J281/Fr341). Simultaneously, the poems exude a daring, irreverent tone and a fearlessness in asking unasked questions, exploring the newly perceived idea of death outside the framework of religious consolation, our darkest, our ultimate fears. This is her great gift to us, a willingness to think through and express these previously inexpressible, unexpressed states in a poetry of affective thought.

Dickinson, of course, had found her way through these horrors very early, as evidenced in the great poems celebrating transience that occur throughout her corpus side by side with the poems of torment and pain—poems such as "These are the days when Birds come back" (J130/Fr122), "I dreaded that first Robin, so" (J348/Fr347), "It bloomed and dropt, a Single Noon" (J978/Fr843), "That it will never come again / Is what makes life so sweet" (J1741/Fr1761)— which make it clear that it was her choice, rather than some uncontrollable psychic compulsion, to explore and give voice to these turbulent psychic states associated with death and mourning. In these poems that celebrate the fact that "Changelessness is Nature's change" (L948), there is an affirmation and an embrace of transience. There is an intrinsic acknowledgment that loss and mourning are "the necessary suffering that makes more life possible" and that "refusal to mourn is refusal to live."[9]

We also have the testament of Dickinson's letters to her friends, which are among the great letters of literature, and many of them are "texts of mourning" comparable in grace and insight to Jacques Derrida's great eulogies to his friends and colleagues, collected in his recent book, *The Work of Mourning*. If Dickinson's death poems give us the gothic Freudian scene, her letters give us the Derridean scene. In both, she is the philosophical friend with and through whom we may think through our own relations to death, to our specific dead, to the beloved dead. What we learn from Derrida—and Dickinson—is that true mourning involves an acceptance of incomprehension. Derrida rejects the Freudian schema as well as that of Abraham and Torok. He argues that we do not need to abandon our dead, and that we can have an ongoing relationship with them through an active, future-oriented remembrance. In fact, he asserts, it is through our active remembrance—our ongoing conversation with the dead—that true mourning occurs.

In 1986, Derrida published a very beautiful book on memory and mourning for his friend Paul de Man, who died in 1984. In *Memoires for Paul de Man*, Derrida abandons the classical terminology of mourning, replacing it with a concept refracted through Hegel and Heidegger of a future-oriented, constitutive, thinking memory (he uses the German word *Gedächtnis* to specify his concept) in which the other now exists simultaneously within us but beyond us. On the death of the other, we are left with traces and fragments of them—their words and ideas and projects, images and representations, the sound of their voice, their look—in "a memory which suddenly seems greater and older than us," "sublimely greater" with this other as other who is now a part of us "in and beyond mournful memory." "To this thought," he writes, "there belongs the gesture of faithful friendship, its immeasurable grief, but also its life: the sublimity of a mourning without sublimation and without the obsessive triumph of which Freud speaks."[10] There is a sense in Derrida, as in Dickinson, that we are "mentally permanent" and that "'It is finished' can never be said of us"(L555).[11]

In *The Work of Mourning,* Derrida depathologizes mourning and finds in it the beauty of friendship and of our connection with some kind of beyond—he calls it "infinite alterity."[12] Dickinson has a similar sense of infinity in the presence of death. Writing to her friend and mentor Thomas Wentworth Higginson on the death of his baby daughter, she says in her distinctive way, "These sudden intimacies with Immortality, are expanse—not Peace—as Lightning at our feet, instills a foreign Landscape" (L641). Derrida says that all our relationships are, from the beginning, tinged with mourning because the unspoken truth of every relationship is that one of us will live to see the other die. All our relationships are tinged with the presence of death and we fail to live fully if we forget this. Derrida also says that we are who we are because of the memory, or more actively, because of our remembrance of those whom we have loved and whom we carry within us. In a sense, "to be" is also "to be haunted." We come into being in dialogue with our dead and can only think of ourselves in "bereaved allegory."[13] Derrida describes it in the following way: "This terrible solitude which is mine or ours at the death of the other is what constitutes that relationship to self, which we call 'me.'"[14] For Derrida, mourning is constitutive; it is the memory of the future death of the other that constitutes our interiority.

When the death of a friend occurs, the friend exists within us, but where classic psychoanalysis has said that we must evict this uncanny tenant, Derrida, like Dickinson, says that we remain in dialogue with him or her and thereby "dialecticize death."[15] In this dialogue, we find expanse. The dead are both within us and between us but also beyond us. And it is because the dead are both beyond us as "infinite alterity" and in us that we gain our experience of infinity and of the beyond. It is this that makes sense of the many times in the poems and letters when Dickinson links the idea of death with the idea of God, as, indeed, does Derrida in his later writing. For both Dickinson and Derrida the loss of a loved one is the loss of a world: "Forgive the Tears that fell for few, but that few too many, for was not each a World?" (L890) writes Dickinson, while Derrida says that in each death there is "another end of the world."[16] Nevertheless, it is death that creates a space for the idea of infinity. Death in Dickinson is the beyond made luminous by love.

In the presence of death, Dickinson is a wise companion; no one has written so much about death and dying—and the difficult fact of remaining behind. Many of her contemporaries learned this about her. "The Wilderness is new— to you. Master let me lead you," she wrote to Higginson on the death of his wife in 1877, enclosing the lines,

> Perhaps she does not go so far
> As you who stay — suppose —
> Perhaps comes closer, for the lapse
> Of her corporeal clothes — (L517; J1399/Fr1455)

And later, she assures him, "Dear friend, I think of you so wholly that I cannot resist to write again, to ask if you are safe? Danger is not at first, for then we are unconscious, but in the after—slower—Days. . . . Love is it's own rescue, for we—at our supremest, are but it's trembling Emblems" (L522).

There are perhaps no letters more beautiful than those Dickinson wrote to her beloved friend Samuel Bowles, editor of the *Springfield Daily Republican*, who, as his obituary stated, though married, "loved and was loved by a num-ber of 'good women,' of the highest intellectual grade."[17] Dickinson was one of these women. In 1877, the year before Bowles died, Dickinson wrote a letter to him in which she enclosed a poem.

> I have no Life but this —
> To lead it here —
> Nor any Death — but lest
> Dispelled from there —
> Nor tie to Earths to come —
> Nor Action new
> Except through this extent
> The love of you. (L515; J1398/Fr1432)

When Bowles died a few months later on January 16, 1878, Dickinson was dev-astated, and in extravagant, heartfelt letters to his wife and to other friends, she left a beautiful, poignant record of mourning. She wrote immediately, on the day of his death, to his wife, Mary Bowles: "To remember our own Mr Bowles is all we can do" (L532), later thanking her: "To be willing that I should speak to you was so generous, dear. . . . Love makes us 'heavenly' without our trying in the least. . . . Dear 'Mr. Sam' is very near, these midwinter days. When purples come on Pelham, in the afternoon we say 'Mr. Bowles's colors'" (L536). In late summer 1878, she reassures Mary that she will never be forgotten: "To forget you would be impossible, had we never seen you; for you were his for whom we moan while consciousness remains. As he was himself Eden, he is with Eden, for we cannot become what we were not" (L567). She also confided to her friend Sophia Holland in the spring of l878: "They say that God is everywhere, and yet we always think of Him as somewhat of a recluse. . . . It is hard not to hear again that vital 'Sam is coming'—though if grief is a test of a priceless life, he is compensated. . . . 'This tabernacle' is a blissful trial, but the bliss predominates" (L551).

Shortly after Bowles's death, Dickinson also initiated a correspondence with Maria Whitney, another of his intellectual friends, acknowledging their shared love: "Dear friend, I have thought of you often since the darkness,—though we cannot assist another's night" (L537)—"To relieve the irreparable degrades it" (L538). In late 1878 she writes to Whitney, "I hope that you are well, and in full receipt of the Great Spirit whose leaving life was leaving you" (L573). In early 1879, she wrote,

> We cannot believe for each other—thought is too sacred a despot, but I hope that God, in whatever form, is true to our friend. . . . Consciousness is the only home of which we *now* know. . . . When not inconvenient to your heart, please remember us, and let us help you carry it, if you grow tired. Though we are each unknown to ourself and each other, 'tis not what well conferred it, the dying soldier asks, it is only the water. (L591)

Dickinson initiates the correspondence with Whitney because of their shared love of Bowles. She offers love and friendship to one she does not know because it is fellowship and creaturely feeling for which we yearn in the presence of death. And it is in this spirit that friendship is proffered and thus, through community with the dead (their shared loved of Bowles), community with the living is born. This act reinforces Judith Butler's idea that grief does not isolate but rather builds a sense of community by foregrounding our relational ties to others. In that sense, "loss makes a tenuous 'we' of us all," and what grief reveals is "the thrall in which our relations with others hold us. . . . We're undone by each other. And if we're not, we're missing something."[18]

The correspondence with Whitney continued until Dickinson's death, demonstrating Bowles's ongoing presence in her life and that of the community of women who shared their love of him: Mary, Maria, and Emily. In 1880, when Whitney moved to Cambridge to live with her brother, Dickinson assures her that she will not be forgotten: "Your name is taken as tenderly as the names of our Birds, or the Flower, for some mysterious cause, sundered from it's Dew — Hoarded Mr Samuel — not one bleat of his Lamb — but is known to us" (L643). Several years later, in 1885, the year before her own death, Dickinson concludes a letter to Whitney with these words: "I fear we shall care very little for the technical resurrection, when to behold the one face that to us comprised it is too much for us, and I dare not think of the voraciousness of that only gaze and its only return. Remembrance is the great tempter" (L969). Later that year, upon seeing a reference in the *Springfield Daily Republican* to a forthcoming biography, *The Life and Times of Samuel Bowles*, she writes ecstatically to Whitney, saying, "I was much quickened toward you and all Celestial things to read (see) that the Life of our loved Mr. Bowles would be with us in Autumn" (L974).

The last decade of Dickinson's life was punctuated by the deaths of those whom she loved. However, reading through the letters of the dying years, I was struck by the fact that, even in the presence of death, she never gives up on life. Far from it, as she writes to Maria Whitney in the summer of 1883.

> You speak of "disillusion." That is one of the few subjects on which I am an infidel. Life is so strong a vision, not one of it shall fail. Not what the stars have done, but what they are to do, is what detains the sky. . . . To have been made alive is so chief a thing, all else inevitably adds. Were it not riddled by partings, it were too divine. (L860)

In late autumn, 1884, she wrote to Nellie Sweetser that "an enlarged ability for missing is perhaps a part of our better growth, as the strange Membranes of the Tree broaden out of sight" (L951). Somewhat more jocularly, she suggests in prose fragment 71 (of the *Letters)* that "did we not find (gain) as we lost we should make but a threadbare exhibition after a few years." She also suggests that "we do not think enough of the Dead as exhilarants — they are not dissuaders but Lures — Keepers of that great Romance still to us foreclosed — while coveting (we envy) their wisdom we lament their silence" (PF50).

There is a sense in these years that Dickinson is both pained and at peace with her dead, that she has achieved a positive relation to them. In late June 1883, she writes to Maria Whitney that "the past is not a package one can lay away. I see my father's eyes, and those of Mr. Bowles — those isolated comets.

If the future is mighty as the past, what may vista be?" (L830). And in a letter to Mary Bowles in June 1882, she recounts a rather tender story of her father feeding the birds in a particularly cold winter. He is no longer the one whose heart is "pure and terrible" (L418), as she had written to Higginson on the occasion of her father's death in 1874, but a loving presence.

> The last April that father lived, lived I mean below, there were several snow-storms, and the birds were so frightened and cold they sat by the kitchen door. Father went to the barn in his slippers and came back with a breakfast of grain for each, and hid himself while he scattered it, lest it embarrass them. Ignorant of the name or fate of their benefactor, their descendants are singing this afternoon.
>
> As I glanced at your lovely gift, his April returned. I am powerless toward your tenderness.
>
> Thanks of other days seem abject and dim, yet antiquest altars are the fragrantest. The past has been very near this week, but not so near as the future — both of them pleading, the latter priceless. (L644)

It is because of her courage and compassion in the exploration of death and grieving that I have come to think of Emily Dickinson as a friend in the sense of a presence that enables us to think about important things in a safe kind of way and to entertain speculations that might otherwise be frightening or overwhelming. Her example of a contemplative, philosophical approach to ideas and experience is enabling and encouraging. In *What Is Philosophy?* Gilles Deleuze and Félix Guattari contend that science deals with prospects, poetry with affects, and philosophy with concepts, and they introduce the idea of the conceptual persona or the philosophical friend who enables thought: "the friend who appears in philosophy no longer stands for an extrinsic persona, an example or empirical circumstance, but rather for a presence that is intrinsic to thought, a condition of possibility of thought itself." They call these "friends" conceptual personae and suggest that the internalized idea of a wise friend "is even said to reveal the Greek origin of philo-sophy."[19] And this is how I have come to think of Emily Dickinson. She is my philosophical friend. Just as she had her "supposed persons" ("When I state myself, as the Representative of the Verse — it does not mean — me — but a supposed person" [L268]) who enabled her to work through her conceptual conundrums, I have my Emily Dickinson. In her capacity as friend and guide, Emily Dickinson also offers a kind of "containment" for the negotiation of violent emotions, and the conversion of fear, loss, and aggression into something that can be named, thought about, or dreamed, and thus transformed.[20] As a conceptual persona, Dickinson allows her readers the space to work through powerful emotions and to transform them. It is because she both acknowledges violent emotion and finds a way through it that she can serve as a kind of holding presence that increases our own capacity for tolerance and thought.

NOTES

1. Judith Butler, *Precarious Life: The Powers of Mourning and Violence* (New York: Verso, 2004), 21.

2. Sigmund Freud, "Mourning and Melancholia," in *On Metapsychology: The Theory of Psychoanalysis*, vol. 11, ed. James Strachey (1917; London: Penguin, 1964), 262.

3. Melanie Klein, "Mourning and Its Relation to Manic-Depressive States," in *The Selected Melanie Klein* (London: Penguin, 1986), 156.

4. Nicolas Abraham and Maria Torok, "Mourning or Melancholia," in *The Shell and the Kernel* (Chicago: Univ. of Chicago Press, 1994), 136.

5. Butler, 46.

6. Ibid., 22.

7. Freud, 252.

8. Ibid., 253.

9. Adam Phillips, *Darwin's Worms* (London: Faber and Faber, 1999), 27.

10. Jacques Derrida, *Memoires for Paul De Man* (New York: Columbia Univ. Press, 1986), 38.

11. Dickinson wrote to Sophia Holland in 1878: "How unspeakably sweet and solemn—that whatever await us of Doom or Home, we are mentally permanent. 'It is finished' can never be said of us" (L555).

12. Jacques Derrida, *The Work of Mourning* (Chicago: Univ. of Chicago Press, 2001), 161.

13. Derrida, *Memoires*, 28.

14. Ibid., 33.

15. Derrida, *Work of Mourning*, 50.

16. Ibid., 95.

17. Jay Leyda, *The Years and Hours of Emily Dickinson* (New Haven, Conn.: Yale Univ. Press, 1960), 286.

18. Butler, 22–23.

19. Gilles Deleuze and Félix Guattari, *What Is Philosophy?* (London: Verso, 1994), 2–3.

20. Julia Segal, *Melanie Klein* (London: Sage, 1992), 122.

"Myself — the Term between —"

Roland Hagenbüchle

Many of Dickinson's poems begin innocently enough as homely analogies or metaphors and then suddenly expand into dazzling symbols, opening up vast spaces of possibility: infinity, eternity, immortality. These broad concepts that she manages to wield in ways unsurpassed in poetic writing make us acutely aware that the lives we normally lead are a degraded version of the real thing—of our true and innermost potential.

To our everyday world of narrow materialism, Dickinson offers in opposition a richly symbolic universe. Against the male fantasy of ruthless force and technocratic hubris, she sets the ecstatic power of poetic imagination, uniquely capable of bridging the here and hereafter thus adding a transcendent dimension to our existence, without which life would become weightless and stale. "That we are of the sky" (J1643/Fr1682), as she wryly puts it, is Dickinson's "Pierless Bridge" (J915/Fr978), a faith always threatened by doubt but one that she stubbornly clings to throughout her life. It is the "angel art" with which she never ceases to wrestle; it is her royal dominion, consecration, and torment in one, a presence both feared and desired, the cause of all her anguish and her ecstasy.

That the *angelus artis* is at the same time the *angelus mortis,* and that the poet's wrestling with the angel art is a fight to the death, no attentive reader of her poems will seriously doubt. Hence, the thanato-erotic anxiety that pervades all her life and work. In order to outmatch the "Bisecting / Messenger" (J1411/Fr1421), death, she pitches Thanatos against Eros, forcing the mighty angel to bless her: "Poetry — // Or Love — the two coeval come" (J1247/Fr1353). It is Dickinson's deep strategy to reverse life's ineluctable depletion into "sumptuous destitution."[1] In this way, she succeeds in keeping mortality and loss at a distance. Through her art, she masters both. Whether Dickinson could have

All citations of Dickinson's poems used in this chapter are from *The Poems of Emily Dickinson,* ed. R. W. Franklin, 3 vols. (Cambridge, Mass.: Harvard Univ. Press, 1998).

survived without the resources of her creative genius is a question I dare not approach. "That we are of the sky" (J1643/Fr1682) remains for us the continuing provocation of Emily Dickinson's incomparable art; it is the clarion call that, however muted at times, echoes through her poetry and will keep echoing through the centuries. We feel impoverished by her riches yet enriched in our poverty through the example of her life and work.

NOTES

This is the text of Roland Hagenbüchle's response (in absentia) to receiving the honor of the Emily Dickinson International Society Distinguished Service Award in August 2004.

1. Roland Hagenbüchle, "Sumptuous Destitution: The Function of Desire in Emily Dickinson's Poetry," *The Emily Dickinson Journal* 5.2 (1996): 1–9.

Dare you see a soul at the "White Heat"?

I began reading Emily Dickinson as an adolescent, and have continued throughout my life; her work retains, for me, the drama and "white-hot" intensity of adolescence, like the work of Henry David Thoreau. Certain of Dickinson's poems are very likely more deeply imprinted in my soul than they were ever imprinted in the poet's, and inevitably reside more deeply, and more mysteriously, than much of my own work.

Dickinson never shied away from great subjects of human suffering: loss, death, even madness, but her perspective was intensely private; like Rainer Maria Rilke and Gerard Manly Hopkins, she is the great poet of inwardness, of that indefinable region of the soul in which we are, in a sense, all one.

JOYCE CAROL OATES
From her introduction to *The Essential Emily Dickinson* (1996)

Contributors

ELLEN BACON is the widow of Pulitzer Prize–winning American composer Ernst Bacon (1898–1990), with whom she spent the last two decades of his life in Orinda, California. Ernst Bacon is especially known for his sixty-seven-song settings of Emily Dickinson's poems. Believing that his affinity to Dickinson was like that of Schumann for Heine, he wrote that she could, "with an economy as great as the classical Chinese poets and painters, conjure ecstasy, poignancy, immensity, grief, passion, and intimacy with nature." Mrs. Bacon is president of the Ernst Bacon Society and teaches piano at her home in Syracuse, New York.

BRUCE BODE is a Unitarian minister at Quimper Unitarian Universalist Fellowship in Port Townsend, Washington. His theological perspective as a naturalist-mystic has been influenced by such figures as Albert Schweitzer, Carl Jung, and poets Mary Oliver, Robert Bly, and Emily Dickinson.

BARBARA DANA is an award-winning author of books for children and young adults. Her books include *Zucchini* (1982), *Zucchini Out West* (1997), *Crazy Eights* (1981), *Necessary Parties* (1986), and *Young Joan* (1991), based on the life of Joan of Arc. She co-wrote the screen version of her novel *Necessary Parties,* aired on PBS. Other screenplays include *Chu Chu and the Philly Flash* and the short film *T.G.I.F.,* honored at the New York Film Festival. Her first play, *War in Paramus,* premiered off-Broadway at the Abingdon Theatre Company in 2005. She is an actor as well as an author, having appeared on Broadway, in films, and on television since the age of sixteen. Barbara is currently working on a novel for HarperCollins based on the young life of Emily Dickinson.

ELLEN LOUISE HART lives in Portland, Oregon, where she is currently writing about the prosody of Dickinson's letters and verse. She is co-editor of *Open Me Carefully: Emily Dickinson's Intimate Letters to Susan Huntington Dickinson* (1998) and associate editor of the Dickinson Electronic Archives. She has published articles on reading Dickinson's manuscripts and has served on the board of the Emily Dickinson

International Society since 1995. She taught for twenty-two years at the University of California at Santa Cruz.

ROLAND HAGENBÜCHLE was sponsored by the American Council of Learned Societies as a postdoctoral fellow at Yale University. There he became friends with renowned Dickinson scholar and biographer Richard Sewall, with whom he shared a love of Dickinson's writings. He is American Council Professor Emeritus of American Studies at the Catholic University of Eichstätt and author of *Emily Dickinson Wagnis der Selbstbegnung.*

CYNTHIA HOGUE is a Maxine and Jonathan Marshall Chair in Modern and Contemporary Poetry at Arizona State University, where she is also director of the Creative Writing Program. She has published four collections of poetry, including *Flux* (2002) and *The Incognito Body* (2006), and her critical work includes the first edition of H.D.'s *The Sword Went Out to Sea* (2007). Among her honors are NEA and Fulbright fellowships and the 2004–5 H.D. Fellowship at the Beinecke Library at Yale University. She has published a range of critical and creative works on Emily Dickinson.

JOAN KIRKBY is a professor in the Department of Critical and Cultural Studies at Macquarie University in Sydney, Australia. She is on the editorial board of the *Emily Dickinson Journal.* She is currently working on three projects on Dickinson: *Emily Dickinson and Evolutionary Theology; Emily Dickinson's Debate with the Nineteenth-Century Philosophical Tradition,* an ARC Large Grant project that examines Dickinson's writing in the context of nineteenth-century periodical literature; and *The Emily Dickinson Compendium.*

JOY LADIN holds the David and Ruth Gottesman Chair in English and directs the Writing Center at Stern College of Yeshiva University. She has also taught writing and literature at Reed College, Princeton University, and the University of Massachusetts at Amherst. In 2002 she served as poet in residence at Tel Aviv University on a Fulbright Scholarship. Several of her critical essays have appeared in the the *Emily Dickinson Journal,* and she is a regular contributor to *Parnassus: Poetry in Review.* Her first collection of poems, *Alternatives to History,* was published in 2003. Her poems have appeared in many magazines and journals, including *New Writing, North American Review, Storie,* and *American Literary Review.* With the assistance of a fellowship from the American Council of Learned Societies, she is currently completing a critical study of the emergence of American modernist poetics between 1850 and 1920.

POLLY LONGSWORTH is author of *The World of Emily Dickinson* (1990) and *Austin and Mabel: The Amherst Affair and Love Letters of Austin Dickinson and Mabel Loomis Todd* (1984). She is a contributing essayist to *The Dickinsons of Amherst* and is currently at work on a new biography of Emily Dickinson. She serves on the board of governors of the Emily Dickinson Museum in Amherst.

CINDY MACKENZIE teaches English at the University of Regina in Regina, Saskatchewan, Canada. She has written both a master's thesis (1988) and a doctoral dissertation (1997) on Emily Dickinson's language, and her articles appear in the *Emily Dickinson Bulletin* and the *Emily Dickinson Journal*. She is the author of *A Concordance to the Letters of Emily Dickinson* (2000) and serves on the board of the Emily Dickinson International Society. She is currently writing a book-length study of Dickinson's use of rhetorical devices titled "'To Pile Like Thunder': Emily Dickinson's Poetics" and is associate editor of a collection of essays on Dickinson's letters.

MELL MCDONNELL began her career as a teacher of English at the University of Cincinnati and the University of New Orleans, where she taught drama, poetry, and writing. She then worked for fifteen years as a public relations/marketing writer and consultant in the financial industry. In 1982 Mell fell in love with the Colorado Shakespeare Festival when she moved from New Orleans to Colorado. A long-term festival volunteer and twice president of the Colorado Shakespeare Guild, she is now marketing and public relations director for the festival.

GREGORY ORR is the author of *Poetry As Survival* (2002) and a memoir, *The Blessing* (2002), as well as nine collections of poems, the most recent of which is *Concerning the Book That Is the Body of the Beloved* (2005). He is professor of English at the University of Virginia and has been the recipient of Guggenheim and NEA fellowships and an Award in Literature from the American Academy of Arts and Letters.

LINDA RICHARD is a writer who has had a long career in journalism and filmmaking. She lives in San Francisco.

MARTHA NELL SMITH is a professor of English and founding director of the Maryland Institute for Technology in the Humanities (MITH) at the University of Maryland, College Park. Author of the award-winning *Rowing in Eden: Rereading Emily Dickinson* (1992), Smith is the coauthor of *Comic Power in Emily Dickinson* (1993) and *Open Me Carefully: Emily Dickinson's Intimate Letters to Susan Huntington Gilbert* (1998). She is the coordinator and executive editor of the Dickinson Electronic Archives Project (http://emilydickinson.org).

MARION WOODMAN is well-known as an international lecturer and workshop leader. Her first career was as a high school teacher of English and creative theater. Her love of literature and the arts took her into the study of dreams and the creative process that is constantly at work in the unconscious. After her graduation from the C. G. Jung Institute in Zurich, Switzerland, in 1979, she returned to Toronto, Canada, and focused her practice on addictions and the power of metaphor in understanding addictive behavior. She is the author of several books and tapes, among them *Addiction to Perfection* (1982), *The Pregnant Virgin* (1985), *The Ravaged Bridegroom* (1990), *Leaving My Father's House* (1992), and *Dancing in the Flames* (1996).

Index to Poems Cited

The index uses the first lines of the poems as they appear in *The Poems of Emily Dickinson*, ed. R. W. Franklin, 3 vols. (Cambridge, Mass.: Harvard Univ. Press, 1998).